CANCER CARE PROTOCOLS
For Hospital and Home Care Use

Second Edition

Doris N. Ahana, R.N., M.S.
Marilyn M. Kunishi, R.N., M.S.

Springer Publishing Company
New York

Copyright © 1986 by Springer Publishing Company, Inc.

All rights reserved

No part of this publication may be reproduced, stored in a retrieval system, or transmitted in any form or by any means, electronic, mechanical, photocopying, recording, or otherwise, without the prior permission of Springer Publishing Company, Inc.

Users of this book may use the Patient Education Sheets herein for use with their own patients. We hereby give permission to photocopy the Patient Education Sheets for the above purpose, provided that such use does not result in financial gain to any person, agency, or institution, or in quantity distribution for teaching purposes.

Springer Publishing Company, Inc.
536 Broadway
New York, New York 10012

86 87 88 89 90 / 5 4 3 2 1

Library of Congress Cataloging-in-Publication Data

Ahana, Doris N.
  Cancer care protocols for hospital and home care use.

  1. Cancer—Nursing—Planning. 2. Medical protocols.
3. Cancer—Patients—Hospital care—Planning. 4. Cancer—
Patients—Home care—Planning. I. Kunishi, Marilyn M.
II. Title. [DNLM: 1. Neoplasms—nursing—handbooks.
2. Nursing Care—standards—handbooks. WY 39 A285c]
RC266.A45 1986   610.73'98   85-30346
ISBN 0-8261-3293-6

Printed in the United States of America

CANCER CARE PROTOCOLS FOR HOSPITAL AND HOME CARE USE

Doris Ahana, R.N., M.S., a former instructor with the School of Nursing at the University of Hawaii, is a clinical nurse specialist in oncology at Saint Francis Hospital in Honolulu, Hawaii. A member of the Oncology Nursing Society, she helped develop Saint Francis Hospital's innovative Cancer Rehabilitation Services (CARES) Program, which combines the expertise of many disciplines in patient rehabilitation. In her capacity as oncology specialist, she integrates and coordinates the delivery of comprehensive care. Ms. Ahana earned her nursing degree at the University of Hawaii and her master's degree in nursing at Wayne State University in Detroit, Michigan. She has contributed to several publications on cancer nursing and is active in community oncology nursing education programs.

Marilyn Kunishi, R.N., M.S., is a clinical nurse specialist at the Veterans Administration Outpatient Clinic in Honolulu, Hawaii. Her responsibilities include coordination of Home Health Services for veterans throughout the state. A nursing graduate of the University of Hawaii, she earned her master's degree in nursing at the University of California, San Francisco Medical Center. She was formerly employed at Saint Francis Hospital, Honolulu, Hawaii as a medical-surgical clinical nurse specialist and was a liaison nurse for the inpatient and home care components of the Cancer Rehabilitation Services (CARES) program. She is an enterostomal therapy graduate of the Cleveland Clinic and is currently an enterostomal consultant to community hospitals.

*To Sister Maureen Keleher, R.N., F.A.C.H.A.,
whose continued support made this revision possible*

"We build on the shoulders of giants"
— R.K. Merton

CONTENTS

Preface   *xvii*
Consultants   *xix*

Part One. GENERAL PROTOCOLS FOR HOSPITAL AND HOME CARE

1. Aging   3

Noncompliance with drug regimen	4
Sensory-perceptual alteration	5
Alteration in nutrition, less than body requirements	6
Ineffective individual coping	8
Impaired physical mobility	10

2. Bone Metastasis   11

Alteration in comfort, pain	12
Impaired physical mobility	13
Potential for injury, pathologic fractures	14
Potential for injury, hypercalcemia	15
Patient Education Sheet 2-1: Exercises for Bedfast Patients	16
Patient Education Sheet 2-2: Transfer Techniques	19

3. Chemotherapy   23

Knowledge deficit	25
Activity intolerance	26

viii Contents

Potential for injury, infection	27
Potential for injury, bleeding	29
Potential for injury, tissue damage	30
Alteration in comfort, joint pain	31
Alteration in oral mucous membrane	32
Alteration in nutrition, less than body requirements, related to nausea and vomiting	33
Alteration in bowel elimination	35
Alteration in self-concept, related to alopecia	36
Nursing Reference 3-1: Cost of Chemotherapeutic Drugs	37
Patient Education Sheet 3-1: Prevention of Bleeding	38
Patient Education Sheet 3-2: Hyperuricemia	41
Patient Education Sheet 3-3: Stomatitis (Sores on Lips, Mouth, or Throat)	43
Patient Education Sheet 3-4: Nausea and Vomiting	47
Patient Education Sheet 3-5: Diarrhea	50
Patient Education Sheet 3-6: Alopecia (Hair Loss)	53
Nursing Reference 3-2: Chemotherapeutic Side Effects and Drug Toxicities	55
Nursing Reference 3-3: Chemotherapy Delivery Systems	59

4. Finances — **61**

Anxiety	62
Knowledge deficit	63
Patient Education Sheet 4-1: Financial Resources	64
Nursing Reference 4-1: Medical Payment Resources	66
Patient Education Sheet 4-2: Financial and Legal Affairs	67

5. Grief — **71**

Grieving, related to cancer diagnosis	72
Ineffective individual coping	74
Ineffective family coping	76
Fear	77
Grieving, related to impending death	78

Contents ix

6. Nutrition 81

Alteration in nutrition, less than body requirements,
  related to treatment modalities, disease process 82
Alteration in nutrition, less than body requirements,
  related to nausea and vomiting 84
Alteration in nutrition, less than body requirements,
  related to diarrhea 85
Alteration in nutrition, less than body requirements,
  related to changes in taste sensation 86
Alteration in nutrition, less than body requirements,
  related to stomatitis or esophagitis 87

Nursing Reference 6-1: Supplements 88
Patient Education Sheet 6-1: Foods Tolerated
  When Nauseous 92
Patient Education Sheet 6-2: Diarrhea Diet 93
Patient Education Sheet 6-3: Food Substitutions
  for Altered Taste Sensation 95
Patient Education Sheet 6-4: Bland Diet 97

7. Oral Care 99

Knowledge deficit 100
Alteration in oral mucosa 101
Potential for injury, gingival bleeding 103
Potential for injury, radiation caries 104

Patient Education Sheet 7-1: Tooth Brushing,
  Tongue Brushing, and Use of Dental Floss 105
Patient Education Sheet 7-2: Mouthwashes 107
Patient Education Sheet 7-3: Denture Care 108

8. Pain 109

Knowledge deficit 110
Alteration in comfort, inadequate relief 111
Alteration in comfort, pain related to anxiety
  and fears 113
Ineffective individual coping 115
Ineffective family coping 116

x **Contents**

Patient Education Sheet 8-1: Management of
    Side Effects   117
Nursing Reference 8-1: Commonly Used Narcotic
    Analgesics Compared with Morphine   118
Nursing Reference 8-2: Commonly Used
    Adjunctive Agents   119
Nursing Reference 8-3: Pain Assessment   120
Nursing Reference 8-4: Alternative Methods of
    Pain Relief   122

9. Radiation Therapy   **125**

Fears   126
Activity intolerance   128
Alteration in nutrition, less than body requirements   129
Alteration in skin integrity   130
Knowledge deficit, side effects in head and neck
    areas   131
Knowledge deficit, side effects in esophagus/chest
    areas   134
Knowledge deficit, side effects in abdominal areas   136

Nursing Reference 9-1: Community Resources for
    Transportation to Radiation Therapy   138

10. Self-Concept   **139**

Altered self-concept related to change in or loss of
    a body part   140
Altered self-concept related to change in role
    performance   141

Nursing Reference 10-1: Counseling   142

11. Sexuality   **143**

Sexual dysfunction, related to ineffective coping   144
Sexual dysfunction, related to change or loss of
    body part   145

Contents xi

Sexual dysfunction, impotence 146
Sexual dysfunction, related to physical limitations 147
Nursing Reference 11-1: Impact of Illness and Other Treatment Modalities on the Sexuality of the Cancer Patient 148

12. Support System 151

Impaired home maintenance management, related to increased care needs 152
Impaired home maintenance management, related to tenuous support system 153
Impaired home maintenance management, related to care giver fatigue 154

Nursing Reference 12-1: Guidelines for Home Care Services 155
Nursing Reference 12-2: Alternative Facilities for Care 159

Part Two. SITE-SPECIFIC PROTOCOLS FOR HOSPITAL AND HOME CARE

13. Bone Cancer 163

Preoperative preparation 164
Potential for injury 165
Impaired physical mobility 167
Alteration in comfort 169
Disturbance in self-concept 170

Nursing Reference 13-1: Leg Stump with Cast and Pylon Attachment 172
Patient Education Sheet 13-1: Stump Care 173
Nursing Reference 13-2: Phantom Limb Sensation and Pain 174
Nursing Reference 13-3: Stump Wrapping 176

14. Bone Marrow Transplant — 179

Preparation of bone marrow transplant patients	180
Knowledge deficit, high-dose chemotherapy	181
Knowledge deficit, radiation	182
Potential for injury, infection	183
Alteration in nutrition, less than body requirements	185
Potential for injury, bleeding, related to thrombocytopenia	186
Activity intolerance	188
Potential for injury, graft versus host disease	189
Sensory-perceptual alteration	191
Ineffective individual coping	193
Ineffective family coping	194
Patient Education Sheet 14-1: Instructions to Prevent Infection	195
Patient Education Sheet 14-2: Reporting to the Physician	197
Patient Education Sheet 14-3: Bone Marrow Transplant Diet for Home Use	198

15. Brain Cancer — 201

Sensory-perceptual alteration, increased intracranial pressure	202
Impaired verbal communication	203
Potential for injury, seizures	204
Sensory-perceptual alteration, diplopia	205
Impaired physical mobility	206

16. Cancers of the Head and Neck — 207

Preoperative preparation	209
Ineffective airway clearance	210
Knowledge deficit	211
Impaired verbal communication	213
Anxiety	214
Potential for injury, infection	216
Impaired physical mobility	218

Alteration in nutrition, less than body requirements	220
Disturbance in self-concept	222
Noncompliance	224
Nursing Reference 16-1: Humidification	225
Patient Education Sheet 16-1: Tracheostomy Care	226
Patient Education Sheet 16-2: Instructions for Shoulder Care	228
Nursing Reference 16-2: Oral Care after Head and Neck Surgery	230
Nursing Reference 16-3: Information on Speech Therapy Services	231
Nursing Reference 16-4: Types of Alaryngeal Speech	232
Patient Education Sheet 16-3: Payment for Purchase of Artificial Larynges and Speech Therapy Services	234
Patient Education Sheet 16-4: Emergency Medical Identification	235
Nursing Reference 16-5: Diet Instructions	236
Patient Education Sheet 16-5: Tracheostomy Coverings	237
Patient Education Sheet 16-6: Head and Neck Exercises	238
Nursing Reference 16-6: Deficits Caused by Head and Neck Surgery	240
Patient Education Sheet 16-7: Books and Pamphlets for Laryngectomy Patients	242
Nursing Reference 16-7: Augmentative Communication	243
Nursing Reference 16-8: Guidelines for Improving Clarity of Speech	244
Nursing Reference 16-9: Dysphagia Program	245

17. Leukemia 247

Activity intolerance	248
Potential for injury, infection related to immunosuppression	249
Potential for injury, bleeding	250

xiv Contents

Alteration in comfort, joint pain ... 251
Fear ... 252
Patient Education Sheet 17-1: Examples of Over-the-Counter Drugs Containing Aspirin and Ibuprofen ... 253

18. Lung Cancer ... 255

Preoperative preparation ... 256
Impaired gas exchange ... 257
Ineffective airway clearance ... 259
Impaired physical mobility ... 260
Activity intolerance ... 261

Patient Education Sheet 18-1: Pursed-Lip and Abdominal Breathing Exercise ... 262
Nursing Reference 18-1: Chest Percussion ... 263
Patient Education Sheet 18-2: Post-Thoracotomy Exercises ... 264
Nursing Reference 18-2: Care of Chest Tubes ... 266

19. Breast Cancer ... 267

Preoperative preparation ... 269
Potential for injury, serous fluid collection ... 270
Potential for injury, wound infection ... 271
Potential fluid volume excess, lymphedema ... 272
Impaired physical mobility ... 274
Disturbance in self-concept ... 276
Anxiety ... 278
Knowledge deficit ... 279

Patient Education Sheet 19-1: The Jackson-Pratt Drain ... 280
Patient Education Sheet 19-2: Arm Support ... 281
Nursing Reference 19-1: Arm Circumference Measurement ... 282
Patient Education Sheet 19-3: Postoperative Exercises ... 283

Contents xv

Nursing Reference 19-2: Mastectomy Exercises	284
Patient Education Sheet 19-4: Post-Mastectomy Exercises	285
Patient Education Sheet 19-5: Suggestions for Preventing Infection and Swelling of Affected Arm and Hand	290
Patient Education Sheet 19-6: Postural Exercise	291
Patient Education Sheet 19-7: Activity Guidelines for Mastectomy Patients	292
Patient Education Sheet 19-8: Temporary Prosthesis	293
Patient Education Sheet 19-9: Permanent Prosthesis Information	294
Nursing Reference 19-3: Self-Help Programs	295

20. Colon Cancer 297

Preoperative preparation	298
Alteration in bowel elimination	299
Potential for injury, perineal wound infection	301
Potential impairment of skin integrity, related to leakage	302
Knowledge deficit, odor and gas	304
Knowledge deficit, colostomy management	305
Potential impairment of skin integrity, side effects of therapy	307
Disturbance in self-concept	308
Sexual dysfunction	309
Patient Education Sheet 20-1: Pouch Change	310
Nursing Reference 20-1: Irrigation of Colostomy	311
Patient Education Sheet 20-2: Appliance for Transverse Colostomy	313
Patient Education Sheet 20-3: Diet Suggestions for Colostomy Clients	316
Patient Education Sheet 20-4: Financial Reimbursement for Ostomy Supplies	317
Patient Education Sheet 20-5: Colostomy Management	318
Nursing Reference 20-2: Ostomy Club Volunteer Visits	320

21. Bladder Cancer — 321

Alteration in pattern of urinary elimination — 322
Knowledge deficit, ileal conduit care — 324
Potential impairment of skin integrity — 326
Knowledge deficit, odor — 328
Disturbance in self-concept — 329
Sexual dysfunction — 330

Patient Education Sheet 21-1: Ileal Conduit—
  Temporary Pouch Change — 331
Patient Education Sheet 21-2: Application of a
  Permanent Urinary Appliance — 332
Patient Education Sheet 21-3: Ileal Conduit
  Management — 334

22. Prostate Cancer — 337

Preoperative preparation — 338
Fluid volume deficit, bleeding — 339
Alteration in pattern of urinary elimination — 340
Sexual dysfunction related to impotence — 341

Patient Education Sheet 22-1: Perineal Exercises — 342

23. Stomach Cancer — 343

Alteration in nutrition, less than body requirements — 344
Knowledge deficit — 345
Alteration in bowel elimination — 346

PREFACE

Five years have passed since the first edition of *Cancer Care Protocols for Hospital and Home Care Use* was published. In that time, two major developments have influenced the format of this second edition.

The first development is the widespread acceptance of a taxonomy or classification system for nursing diagnoses. This led to the use of nursing diagnoses and outcomes in writing the protocols. Assessment factors have been incorporated into the interventions.

The second development is the advent of Diagnosis Related Groups (DRGs). In an effort to contain costs, the emphasis of care has shifted from the hospital to the home. The site-specific protocols reflect this change. Many interventions previously reserved for the hospital are now more appropriately initiated in the home. That clients are more ill at the time of admission, as well as at discharge, presents a challenge to nurses in both settings. Consistency, continuity, and coordination are essential if this challenge is to be met.

These cancer care protocols are guidelines that delineate basic interventions to achieve desired client outcomes. They encourage the involvement of members of other health disciplines when appropriate, and emphasize the continuum of care from hospital to home. In this text, the protocols are divided into two sections. The general protocols deal with problems common to all cancer patients, such as grief, nutrition, and pain. Site-specific protocols focus on problems caused by cancer in specific areas; for example, the breast or head and neck. References are used to elaborate on interventions that the nurse generalist may not routinely perform. As appropriate, the nursing diagnoses and interventions are identified separately for the hospital and home care settings, or combined when similar. The rationale for interventions is beyond the scope of this book and can be obtained from the many journals and texts on cancer. It is assumed that the practitioner possesses knowledge of the routine postoperative care required by all clients, and of basic nursing procedures and treatments. The authors support the multidisciplinary concept in comprehensive cancer care and encourage nurses using these protocols to utilize the skills of health professionals available to them.

The authors gratefully wish to acknowledge the assistance given us by so many people. The chemotherapy department of St. Francis Hospital allowed us to continue using the teaching tools in the chemotherapy references. Myron Tong, Assistant Administrator, and Florence Aihara, Special Assistant to the Chief Executive Officer, facilitated the technical aspects of producing this revision. Lastly, we would like to thank our families — Mervin, Dori, and Alan Ahana; and Hanayo and Arthur Kunishi — for their patience and support.

CONSULTANTS

The following professionals served as consultants to the authors in the development of protocols in their specialty areas. Their assistance is gratefully acknowledged.

Dianne Fowler, R.P.T., Chief, Department of Physical Therapy, St. Francis Hospital, Honolulu, Hawaii.
(Exercise Programs)

Edward L. S. Jim, M.D., F.A.C.S., head and neck surgeon, Associate Professor of Surgery, School of Medicine, University of Hawaii, Honolulu, Hawaii.
(Head and Neck)

Kathy Kramer, M.S., C.C.S., Sp., R.N., speech–language pathologist, St. Francis Home Care Services, Honolulu, Hawaii.
(Head and Neck)

Thomas K. L. Lau, M.D., internist, Clinical Associate Professor of Medicine, School of Medicine, University of Hawaii, Director of Institute of Oncology, St. Francis Hospital, Honolulu, Hawaii.
(Chemotherapy)

William K. K. Lau, M.D., F.A.C.P., Infectious Disease Chief, Division of Infectious Disease, School of Medicine, University of Hawaii, member of bone marrow transplantation team, St. Francis Hospital, Honolulu, Hawaii.
(Bone Marrow Transplant)

Consultants

Carolyn Mau, R.N., M.S., psychiatric clinical nurse specialist, Pain Treatment Center, St. Francis Hospital, Honolulu, Hawaii.
(Pain)

Carol Murai, R.D., dietitian, St. Francis Home Care Services, Honolulu, Hawaii.
(Nutrition)

Peter G. C. Wong, D.M.D., private practice, Assistant Clinical Professor, Division of Stomatology, School of Medicine, University of Hawaii, Honolulu, Hawaii.
(Oral Care)

Karen Yaji, M.S.W., social worker, Institute of Renal Disease, formerly with Cares-At-Home Program, Honolulu Home Care, St. Francis Hospital, Honolulu, Hawaii.
(Support System, Finances)

Part One
GENERAL PROTOCOLS FOR HOSPITAL AND HOME CARE

Chapter 1
AGING

Noncompliance with drug regimen
Sensory-perceptual alteration
Alteration in nutrition, less than body requirements
Ineffective individual coping
Impaired physical mobility

4 General Protocols

NURSING DIAGNOSIS

Noncompliance, related to lack of knowledge about the use of multiple drugs

OUTCOME

Takes medications correctly

INTERVENTIONS

1. Determine client's compliance with current medication regimen, including over-the-counter drug use.
2. Establish, with the client, a system for taking medications that incorporates his/her daily living pattern. Simplify medication regimen as much as possible.

    - Use medication reminder boxes as needed
    - Schedule pill-taking around mealtimes and waking hours as appropriate
    - Where possible, decrease the number of times routine medications must be taken

3. Instruct family to report changes in behavior activity tolerance, speech and/or gait to the physician or nurse.

NURSING DIAGNOSIS

Sensory-perceptual alterations, related to unfamiliar surroundings, bombardment by multiple stimuli, or deprivation of stimuli

OUTCOME

Demonstrates orientation to reality

INTERVENTIONS

1. Orient to time, place, and person upon each contact.
2. Limit number of staff working with client.
3. Encourage family visits and involvement in care.
4. Maximize interaction and socialization with friends, family, roommate.
5. If isolated, explain reason.
6. Schedule care based upon routines followed by client at home. Involve client in decision making.
7. Assess for visual and hearing deficits. Obtain glasses or hearing aid as needed.
8. Encourage mobilization as tolerated.
9. If necessary, obtain an interpreter to make instructions and concerns clearly understood.

NURSING DIAGNOSIS

Alteration in nutrition, less than body requirements, related to physical or economic constraints secondary to aging and cancer

OUTCOMES

Reports increase in amount of food intake
Utilizes community resources

INTERVENTIONS

1. Assess:

   - Caloric intake, by doing a diet recall
   - Practices contributing to malnutrition
   - Physical deficits that hinder shopping for and preparing meals
   - Financial constraints
   - Bowel irregularities
   - Altered taste sensation
   - Support system

2. Check dentures and bridge for alignment and fit.

3. Refer to community resources such as:

   - Food stamp program
   - Meal delivery programs
   - Senior citizen centers
   - Homemaker services
   - Volunteer/church groups

4. Educate regarding improvement of nutrition, using foods familiar to and affordable by client.

5. Intensify involvement of dietitian during periods of cancer therapy.

Aging 7

6. Consult with physician regarding supplementing diet with vitamins.
7. Consider the use of supplements (Nursing Reference 6-1).

8 General Protocols

NURSING DIAGNOSIS

Ineffective individual coping related to depression in response to cancer being imposed on a pre-existing chronic illness

OUTCOME

Verbalizes feelings and accepts appropriate support

INTERVENTIONS

1. Assess client for symptoms of depression:

    - Change in behavior
    - Fatigue
    - Decreased appetite
    - Sleep disturbance
    - Expression of suicidal thoughts

2. Evaluate strength of client's support system

    - Family involvement with client
    - Friends
    - Church members

3. Utilize support to increase client's participation in activities of daily living.

4. Encourage verbalization of feelings by having one professional primarily involved with client.

5. Make every effort to communicate planned interventions clearly: their purpose and possible side effects. Respect client's right to refuse therapy.

6. Initiate immediate psychiatric intervention if suicidal ideation with a well-planned method of achieving it are verbalized.

7. Refer client/family to community resources such as:

   - Hospice
   - Self-help groups

10 General Protocols

NURSING DIAGNOSIS

Impaired physical mobility, related to decreased strength secondary to aging and cancer

OUTCOME

Maintains optimal function and ability

INTERVENTIONS

1. Obtain baseline measurement of range of motion and activity tolerance.
2. Identify environmental barriers, eliminate safety hazards, and help client/family modify room arrangements as needed.
3. Instruct client and family regarding proper body mechanics.
4. Obtain physical therapy/occupational therapy referral for:

    - Transfer techniques (Patient Education Sheet 2-2).
    - Clients having a mastectomy, thoracotomy, or head and neck surgery
    - Planning of a structured exercise and muscle-strengthening program

5. Assess need for assistive devices. Check appliances client already has for safety of operation.

Chapter 2
BONE METASTASIS

Alteration in comfort, pain
Impaired physical mobility
Potential for injury, pathologic fractures
Potential for injury, hypercalcemia
Patient Education Sheet 2-1: Exercises for Bedfast Patients
Patient Education Sheet 2-2: Transfer Techniques

NURSING DIAGNOSIS

Alteration in comfort: pain, related to bone metastasis

OUTCOME

Expresses relief from pain or increased comfort

INTERVENTIONS

1. Continually evaluate effectiveness of pain medication being prescribed.
2. Assist client and family in setting up a schedule for pain-control drugs.
3. Schedule activities around medication times.
4. Teach client relaxation techniques if guarding or protective body positions increase muscle tension and contribute to disabilities such as contractures.
5. Teach client/family methods of supporting the affected area to minimize pain of transfers. Use orthotics prior to activity as necessary.
6. Check for possible fracture or inflammatory process.
7. Consider use of diversion or referral to a recreational therapist.

NURSING DIAGNOSIS

Impaired physical mobility, related to pain

OUTCOME

Performs activities of daily living

INTERVENTIONS

1. Assess present level of mobility and activity tolerance.
2. Teach client active bed exercise to prevent further deterioration (Patient Education Sheet 2-1).
3. Incorporate "exercises" into daily living routine.
4. Evaluate need for:

    - Assistive devices
    - Referral to physical therapy or occupational therapy

5. Instruct client and family in transfer techniques and body mechanics as needed (Patient Education Sheet 2-2).
6. Assess for areas of potential skin breakdown.

NURSING DIAGNOSIS

Potential for injury, related to pathologic fractures secondary to bone metastasis

OUTCOMES

Demonstrates understanding of need to exercise caution by utilizing correct techniques in activities of daily living
States symptoms of a fracture

INTERVENTIONS

1. Reinforce physician's explanation about areas involved.
2. Instruct client/family about transfer techniques, especially the need to avoid sudden, jarring movements.
3. Caution client about bearing weight on the affected limb, reaching, bending, and lifting. Caution family about pulling on affected extremity.
4. Teach client and family how to recognize a fracture.
5. Establish a safe environment so that client can walk without bumping into objects, sliding on rugs, and so forth.
6. Observe for neurological deficits suggesting spinal cord compression:
   - Back pain
   - Numbness
   - Weakness
   - Alterations in bowel/bladder function

NURSING DIAGNOSIS

Potential for injury, related to hypercalcemia secondary to bone metastasis

OUTCOME

Identifies measures that may decrease serum calcium levels

INTERVENTIONS

1. Encourage mobility to maximum amount tolerable.
2. Monitor serum calcium as ordered by physician.
3. Encourage fluid intake.
4. Teach family symptoms of hypercalcemia when serum calcium is rising:

   - Anorexia
   - Nausea and/or vomiting
   - Constipation
   - Thirst
   - Polyuria
   - Dehydration
   - Confusion
   - Lethargy

5. Review with client and family foods high in calcium and the appropriate use of vitamin D.
6. If client is taking antacids, report to physician use of calcium-containing products (Titralac, Camalox, Dicarbosil).

PATIENT EDUCATION SHEET 2-1
Exercises for Bedfast Patients

Quadriceps Setting

Tighten the kneecap by making the knee stiff. Hold leg stiff for five seconds and relax. Repeat.

Gluteal Setting

Lie with legs out straight. Pretend to pinch a penny between the two buttocks, tightening these muscles. Hold for five seconds and relax. Repeat.

Bridging

1. Bend both knees (Figure 1).

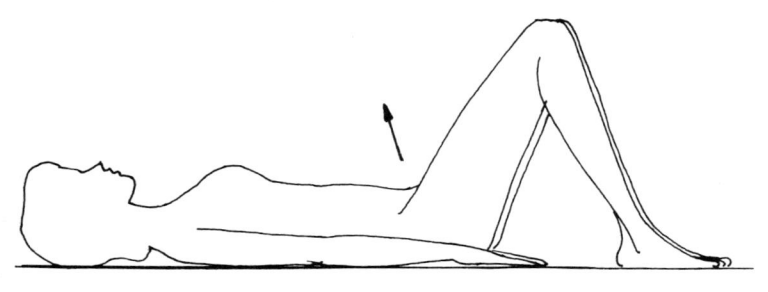

FIGURE 1

2. Raise buttocks off bed to form a straight line from knees to shoulders (Figure 2).

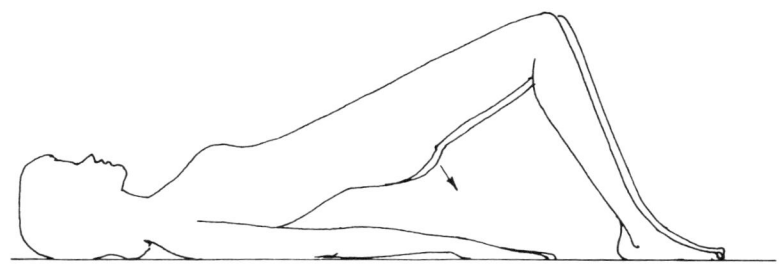

FIGURE 2

3. Hold for five seconds and relax.
4. Repeat.

Shoulder Stretching

Put both hands behind the head and push elbows back against the pillow. Then bring elbows forward across the face. Repeat.

Shoulder Range of Motion

1. Pretend to hold a long stick with both hands across the thighs (Figure 3). Raise the stick from the thighs to over the head. Lower stick to thighs. Repeat.

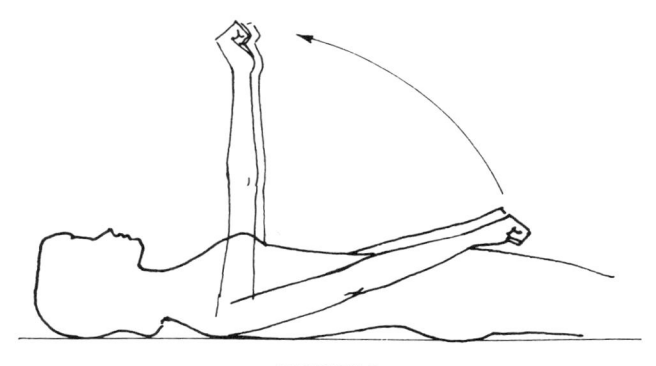

FIGURE 3

18   General Protocols

2. Pretend to hold a long stick with both hands across the chest (Figure 4). Push the stick straight up to the ceiling. Lower the stick. Repeat.

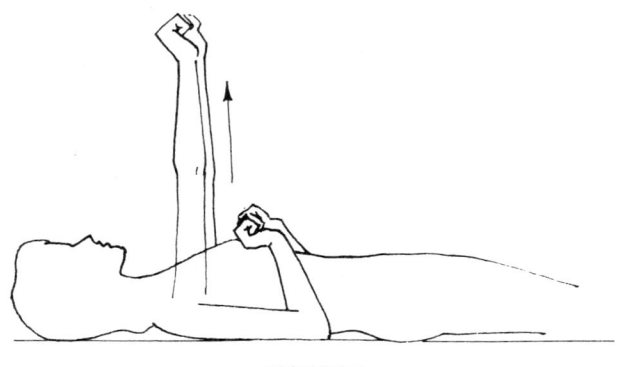

FIGURE 4

PATIENT EDUCATION SHEET 2-2
Transfer Techniques

Lying to Sitting or Standing Position

1. Shift body to the edge of the bed and then turn on the side (Figure 5).

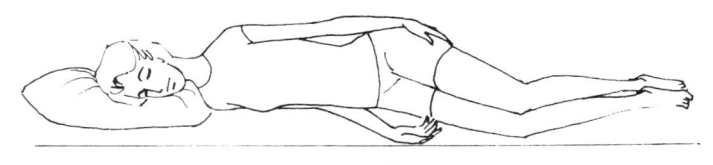

FIGURE 5

2. Using the uppermost arm, push down on the edge of the bed, raising the shoulders and bringing legs off the bed (Figure 6).

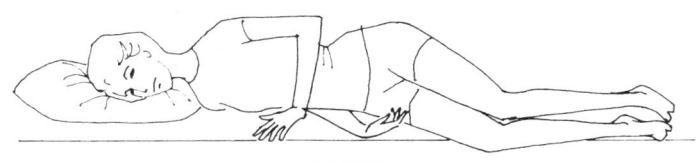

FIGURE 6

3. When the shoulders are off the bed, push down on the elbow closest to the bed for more leverage. Swing legs off the bed completely (Figure 7).

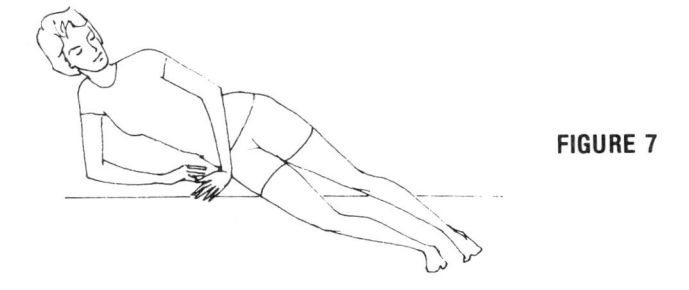

FIGURE 7

4. Place both feet firmly on the floor and straighten up to a standing or sitting position (Figure 8).

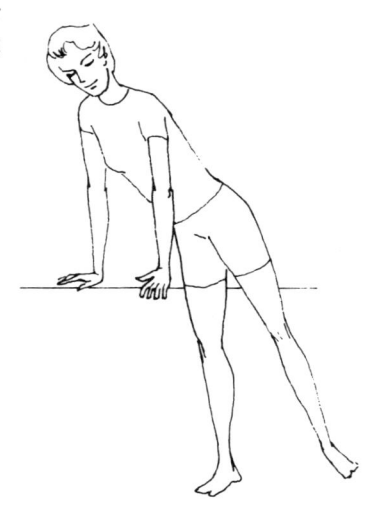

FIGURE 8

Sitting to Standing Position

Position: Sitting erect in chair (Figure 9).

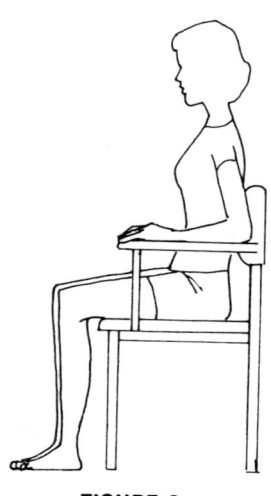

FIGURE 9

1. Slide buttocks to the edge of the chair (Figure 10).

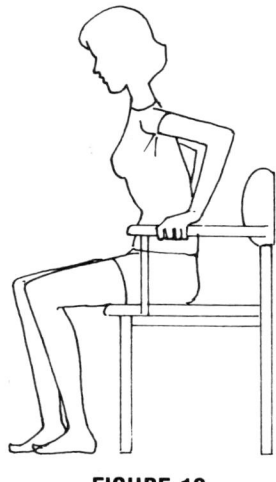

FIGURE 10

22 General Protocols

2. Grasp the arms of the chair firmly and push self up slowly to an upright position (Figures 11 and 12).

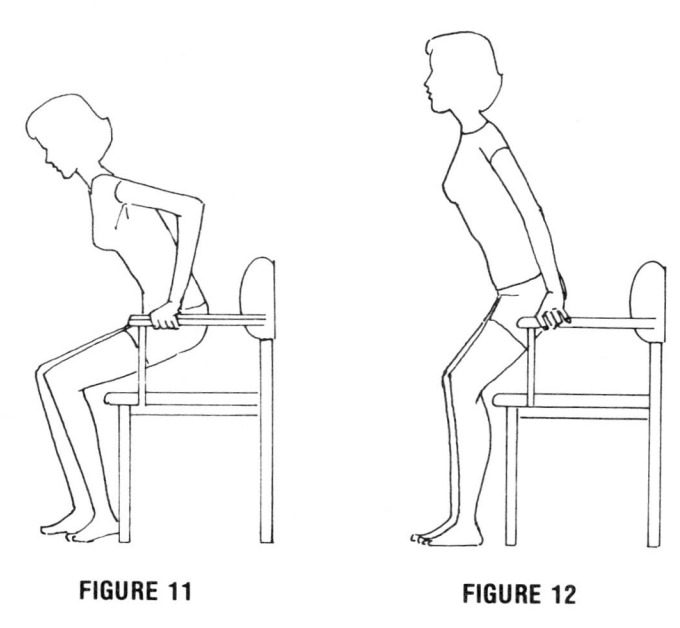

FIGURE 11 **FIGURE 12**

3. Be sure legs and back are straight before walking.

NURSING DIAGNOSIS

Knowledge deficit, related to chemotherapy administration

OUTCOME

Verbalizes understanding of purpose of chemotherapy, route of administration, its side effects, cost

INTERVENTIONS

1. Instruct client and family regarding:

   - Purpose of therapy
   - Route of administration (Nursing Reference 3-3).
   - Scheduling of chemotherapy
   - Type of chemotherapeutic agents used
   - Setting where chemotherapy will be given

2. Forewarn client/family about the possibility of side effects. Explain importance of reporting symptoms (Nursing Reference 3-2).

3. Correct misconceptions client and family may have about chemotherapy.

4. Explain need for baseline laboratory and x-ray studies.

5. Provide information regarding reimbursement of drug costs (Nursing Reference 3-1).

6. Instruct regarding need for optimum nutrition (Nutrition Protocol, Chapter 6).

7. Encourage dental prophylaxis prior to first treatment.

8. Assess mode of transportation, involving family and community agencies as appropriate.

9. As appropriate, reassure regarding symptom management.

NURSING DIAGNOSIS

Activity intolerance, related to fatigue and generalized weakness secondary to anemia induced by chemotherapy

OUTCOMES

Demonstrates techniques to conserve energy
Identifies iron-rich foods

INTERVENTIONS

1. Explain reason for decreased activity tolerance. Reassure that this is a temporary side effect of chemotherapy.
2. Teach client to:

   - Space activities
   - Plan for rest periods
   - Change positions slowly
   - Make transportation arrangements as needed

3. Encourage intake of iron-rich foods. Obtain referral to dietitian if intake is poor.
4. Discuss with family ways they can relieve the client of some of his/her usual household responsibilities.
5. As appropriate, counsel client to discuss work schedule modification with employer.

NURSING DIAGNOSIS

Potential for injury, infection, related to immunosuppression and debilitation secondary to chemotherapy

OUTCOME

Identifies ways to decrease risk of infection

INTERVENTIONS

1. Monitor closely for signs and symptoms of infection:

   - White blood cell count
   - Temperature
   - Alteration in usual respiratory pattern
   - Integrity of skin and mucous membranes
   - Changes in urine color, odor, frequency
   - Erythema induration or drainage at intravenous or intramuscular injection sites

2. Explain and reinforce reason for increased risk of infection.

3. Assess life-style patterns in regard to hygiene. Correct unsafe practices.

4. Instruct regarding need for daily care of:

   - Mouth (Oral Care Protocol, Chapter 7).
   - Skin
   - Genitourinary tract

5. Identify and eliminate environmental risks for infection.

6. Explain need to avoid crowds and people with respiratory infections, herpes zoster, chicken pox.

7. Minimize number of intrusive procedures and *use strict asepsis.*

8. Confer with physician about advisability of immunization against flu and pneumococcal pneumonia.

NURSING DIAGNOSIS

Potential for injury, bleeding, related to thrombocytopenia secondary to chemotherapy

OUTCOME

Identifies measures to decrease risk of bleeding

INTERVENTIONS

1. Monitor platelet count and coagulation profiles closely.
2. Explain and reinforce reason for increased risk of bleeding.
3. Teach client bleeding precautions (Patient Education Sheet 3-1).
4. Consult with dietitian or instruct regarding use of a bland diet if upper gastrointestinal bleeding occurs or is imminent.
5. Obtain order for stool softener if constipation is a problem.

NURSING DIAGNOSIS

Potential for injury, tissue damage, related to extravasation of vesicant or irritant drugs

OUTCOME

Experiences minimal tissue damage

INTERVENTIONS

1. Instruct client to report immediately symptoms of pain, burning, erythema, induration.
2. Assess IV blood return
3. Stop infusion of drug immediately. Examples of vesicant and irritant drugs:

    - Vincristine sulfate (Oncovin)
    - Dactinomycin (Actinomycin-D)
    - Nitrogen Mustard (Mustargen)
    - Mithramycin (Mithracin)
    - Mitomycin-C (Mutamycin)
    - Streptozotocin (Zanosar)
    - Vinblastine sulfate (Velban)
    - Doxorubicin hydrochloride (Adriamycin)
    - Daunomycin hydrochloride (Daunorubicin, Rubidomycin)
    - Dacarbazine (DTIC)
    - Carmustine (BCNU)

4. Contact physician immediately for management orders or follow established protocols.
5. Monitor for long-term effects of extravasation-ulceration, necrosis.

Note: Prevention of extravasation by correct administration of drugs is of paramount importance.

NURSING DIAGNOSIS

Alteration in comfort: pain in joints, related to hyperuricemia secondary to chemotherapy

OUTCOME

Express pain relief or increased comfort

INTERVENTIONS

1. Reassure client/family that joint pain is temporary and not related to metastases.
2. Encourage increased fluid intake.
3. Teach client and family about avoiding high purine foods (Patient Education Sheet 3-2).
4. Reinforce reason for taking uricosuric agents on a prophylactic basis.

NURSING DIAGNOSIS

Alteration in oral mucous membrane related to stomatitis

OUTCOME

Expresses pain relief or increased comfort

INTERVENTIONS

1. Assess status of mucous membranes carefully.
2. Explain to client and family the need for proper oral care (Oral Care Protocol, Chapter 7).
3. Teach client to incorporate bland, soft foods into diet (Patient Education Sheet 3-3).
4. Apply local anesthetic as prescribed by physician. Consider use of pain medication prior to meals.

NURSING DIAGNOSIS

Alteration in nutrition: less than body requirements, related to nausea and vomiting

OUTCOMES

Experiences relief of symptoms
Identifies measures to optimize food intake

INTERVENTIONS

1. Administer antiemetic medication routinely and prior to chemotherapy.
2. Evaluate effectiveness of antiemetic drug.
3. Ask client about personal practices that minimize nausea and vomiting and include them in care:

    - Omission of food prior to treatment
    - Eating specific foods
    - Relaxation techniques
    - Antiemetics that have been helpful previously

4. Instruct client to:

    - Take analgesics and antiemetics prior to meals
    - Alter environmental factors that contribute to nausea and vomiting; e.g., odors, cooking
    - Rinse mouth before meals
    - Eat small portions and more frequently (Patient Education Sheet3-4).

5. Schedule chemotherapy to minimize nausea if possible.

6. Explain that nausea and vomiting are temporary and that short-term decreased food intake is not a cause for concern.
7. Consult with dietitian.

NURSING DIAGNOSIS

Alteration in bowel elimination: diarrhea related to chemotherapy

OUTCOME

Reports decrease in number of stools and minimization of discomfort

INTERVENTIONS

1. Instruct client to take antidiarrheal medications as prescribed.
2. Teach client to incorporate constipating, low-roughage foods in diet (Patient Education Sheet 3-5).
3. Encourage increased intake of room-temperature liquids, fluids high in potassium and sodium.
4. Initiate skin care measures for the perineal area.

NURSING DIAGNOSIS

Alteration in self-concept, related to alopecia

OUTCOMES

Verbalizes feelings about impact of hair loss
Participates in usual activities

INTERVENTIONS

1. Institute nursing measures to minimize hair loss:

   - Scalp tourniquet
   - Hypothermia for scalp

2. Teach client that:

   - Hair loss is temporary and regrowth occurs after chemotherapy is stopped
   - Texture and color of hair may change
   - Hair loss may be rapid and extensive

3. Encourage verbalization of feelings regarding the impact of alopecia:

   - Stigma of having cancer
   - Loss of attractiveness
   - Sexuality

4. Suggest that client purchase a wig, scarf or hat prior to hair loss (Patient Education Sheet 3-6).

5. Refer to local American Cancer Society (ACS) unit for assistance with purchase and selection of a wig.

NURSING REFERENCE 3-1
Cost of Chemotherapeutic Drugs

Medicare
1. Covers 100% of the cost of drugs given while hospitalized.
2. Covers partially the cost of outpatient drugs that cannot be self-administered (for example, intramuscular and intravenous medications).

Private Insurance
1. Usually covers 100% of the cost of drugs given while hospitalized.
2. Covers partially, under certain conditions, the cost of oral outpatient drugs as part of Major Medical Benefits.
3. Covers partially, as part of the Major Medical Benefits, the cost of intravenous and intramuscular medications given in a physician's office or clinic.

Special Cancer Insurance
Refer to policy for coverage.

Investigational Protocols
Regional oncology groups may cover the cost of investigational drugs and/or laboratory work.

PATIENT EDUCATION SHEET 3-1
Prevention of Bleeding

1. Observe for blood in urine or stool, for bleeding from the

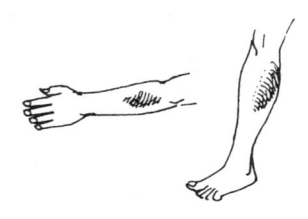

    gum   or the nose

    and for bruises.

Report any signs of bleeding to your physician.

2. Use an electric shaver, not a razor, for shaving.

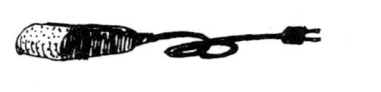

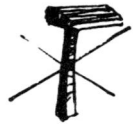

Chemotherapy

3. Good oral care is important. Use soft bristle toothbrush.

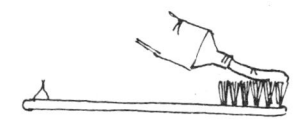

4. Avoid contact sports such as football.

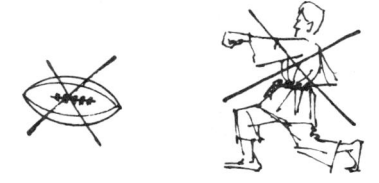

Check with your physician first.

5. Do not take aspirin. Check with your physician first before taking any new medications.

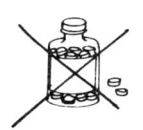

6. Use gloves when you do yard work.

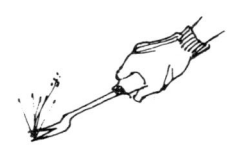

General Protocols

7. If you injure yourself and bleed, apply pressure to area until bleeding stops.

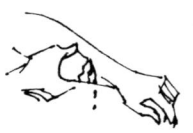

8. Call your doctor for any bleeding that is unusual or that does not stop.

        Physician _____
        Telephone number _____

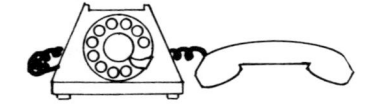

PATIENT EDUCATION SHEET 3-2
Hyperuricemia

Definition: High blood uric acid

1. Tell your physician if you have:

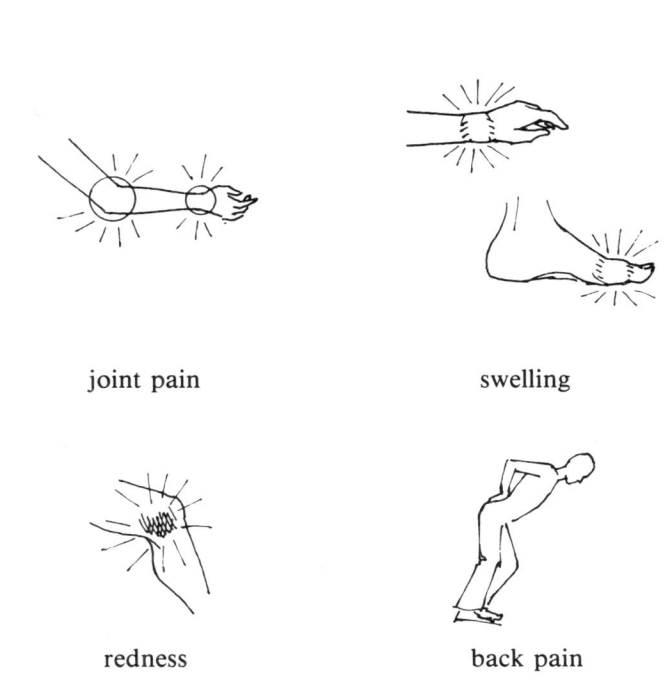

joint pain   swelling

redness   back pain

2. Drink lots of fluids (six to eight cups a day).

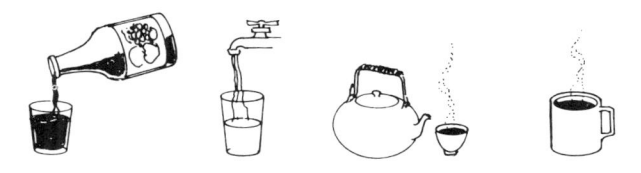

42 General Protocols

3. Foods to limit:

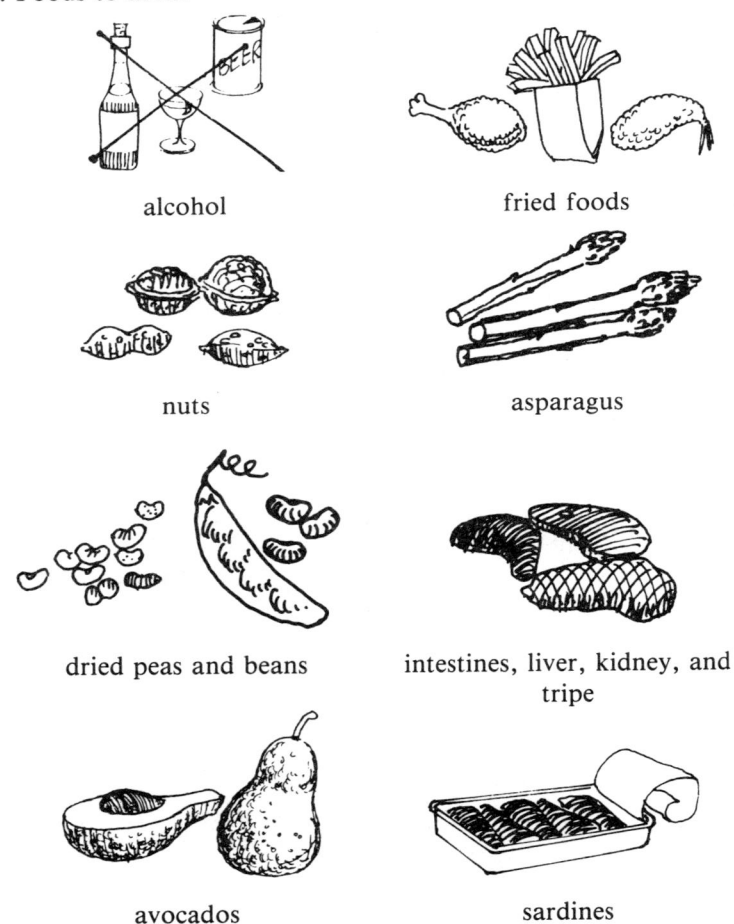

alcohol

fried foods

nuts

asparagus

dried peas and beans

intestines, liver, kidney, and tripe

avocados

sardines

4. Follow the medications prescribed by your doctor.

Drug _____
Instructions _____
Treatment instructions _____

PATIENT EDUCATION SHEET 3-3
Stomatitis (Sores on lips, mouth, or throat)

1. See your dentist for regular checkups.

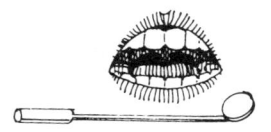

2. Rinse your mouth several times a day with diluted Cepacol, salt water, or a solution of half water and half hydrogen peroxide.

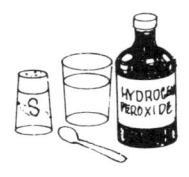

3. Chew Aspergum or suck on hard candy or Cepacol lozenges — this may help to relieve the pain.

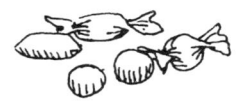

4. If your gums are sore, remove your dentures.

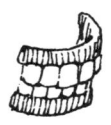

44 General Protocols

5. Take medicines prescribed by your doctor.

Drug _____
Instructions _____
_____

6. Avoid tobacco — it may irritate your gums.

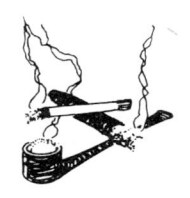

7. Foods to eat:

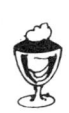

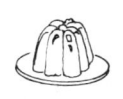

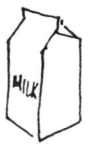

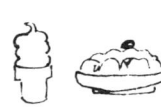

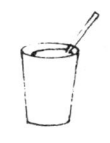

pudding, custard, jello   milk, ice cream, milk shakes

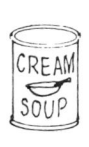

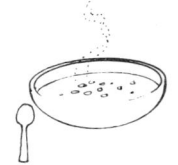

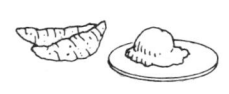

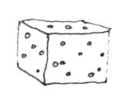

cream   cooked   sweet yams,   soybean
soup   cereals   mashed potatoes,   curd

Chemotherapy 45

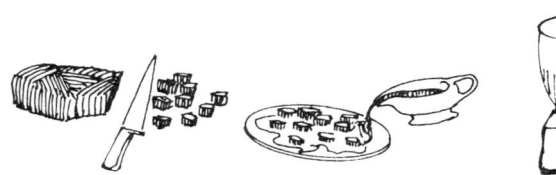

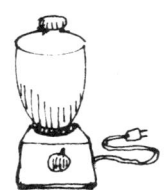

soft meat cut into small pieces with lots of gravy

blenderized foods

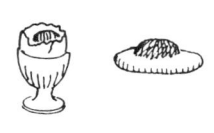

soft or poached eggs

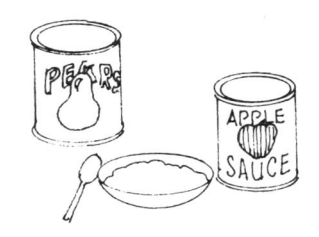

bland canned fruits

8. Foods to avoid:

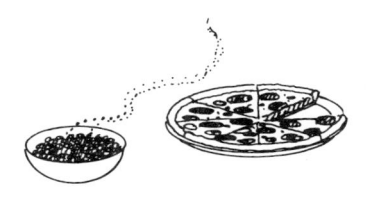

spicy foods

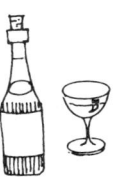

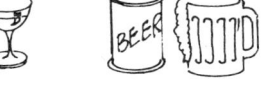

alcoholic beverages

46 General Protocols

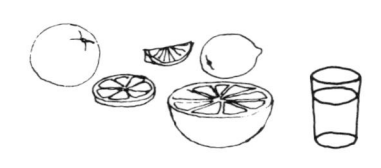

citrus fruits and juices

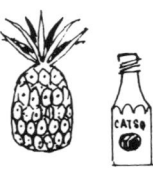

acid foods

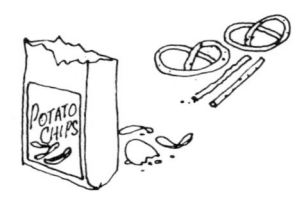

salty foods

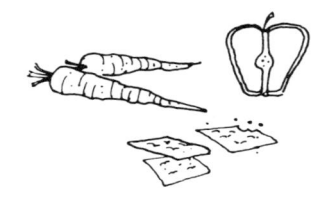

hard foods

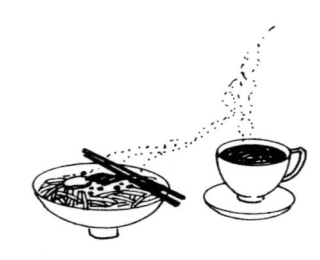

hot foods

PATIENT EDUCATION SHEET 3-4
Nausea and Vomiting

1. Eat lightly before your chemotherapy treatment. Your appetite may not be good after chemotherapy.

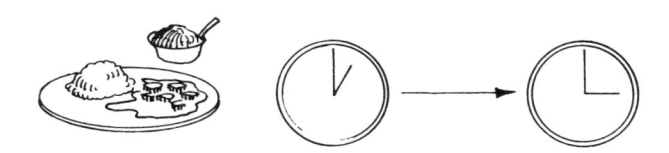

2. Take the medicine prescribed by your doctor.

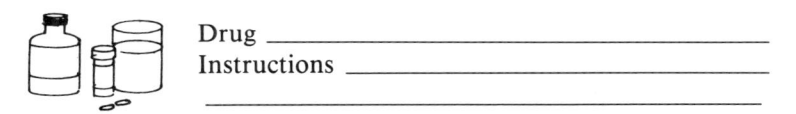

   Drug _____
   Instructions _____
   _____

3. Rinse your mouth with mouthwash or salt water before and after you eat.

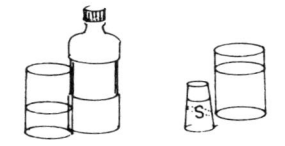

48   General Protocols

4. Avoid things that may make you nauseated — for example, strong smells.

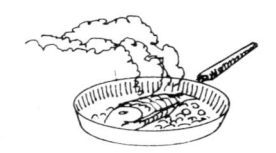

5. Think of ways you controlled nausea before.
6. Ask the dietitian to help you find foods that make you feel less nauseated. Diet siggestions: Eat small amounts of easily digestible foods. You may tolerate five or six small meals better than three large meals.

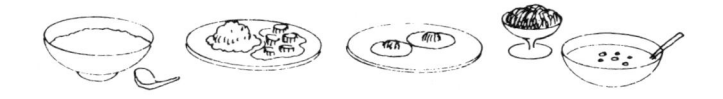

7. Rest and sleep help to minimize the nausea.
8. If these suggestions do not help, call the doctor.
9. Foods to eat:

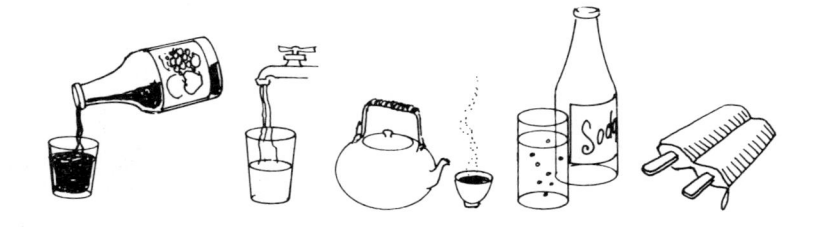

liquids between meals

Chemotherapy 49

crackers and dry toast

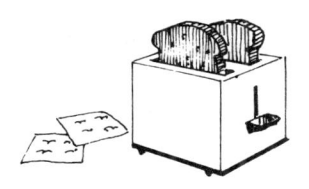

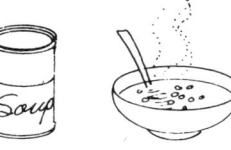

clear soups and broths

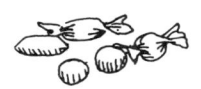

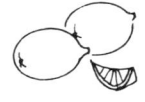

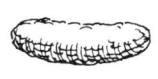

sour candy, lemon, or pickles eaten slowly may help

10. Foods to avoid:

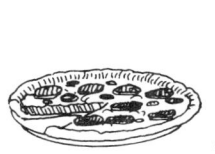

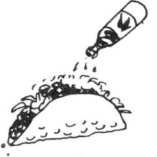

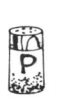

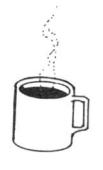

spicy foods and condiments

coffee

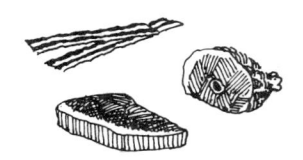

limit bacon, meat, and pork

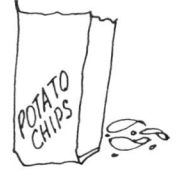

oily foods

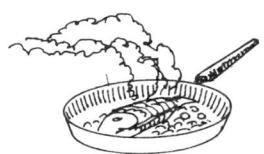

foods with strong odors

50 General Protocols

PATIENT EDUCATION SHEET 3-5
Diarrhea

Definition: Frequent soft or liquid bowel movements

1. Report changes in bowel habits (Figure 13).

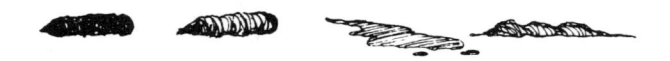

FIGURE 13. BLACK, BLOODY, WATERY, AND SOFT STOOLS.

2. Keep buttock area clean.

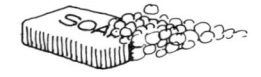

3. Do not smoke or chew tobacco.

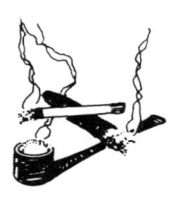

4. Take antidiarrhea drugs prescribed by the doctor.

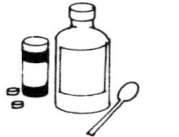

Drug _____
Instructions _____
_____

5. If diarrhea is still not controlled, tell the nurse or doctor.

6. Foods to eat:

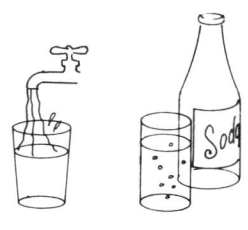

room temperature fluids

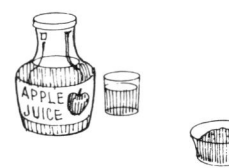

apple juice and apple sauce

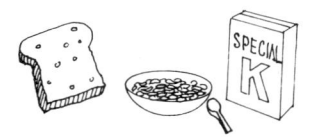

refined bread and cereal

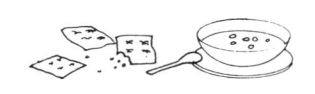

crackers and boullion and consomme broths

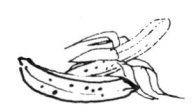

bananas

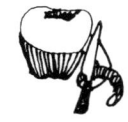

peeled apples

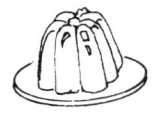

jello

52 General Protocols

7. Foods to avoid:

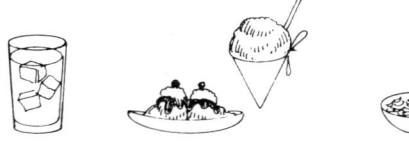

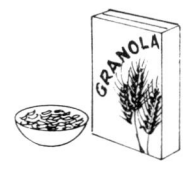

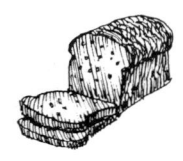

ice cold drinks or foods whole grain cereals and breads

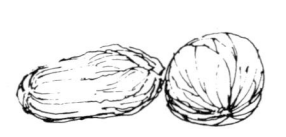

fresh leafy vegetables   fresh fruits   nuts

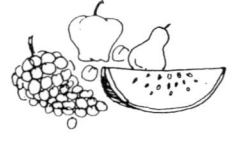

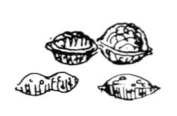

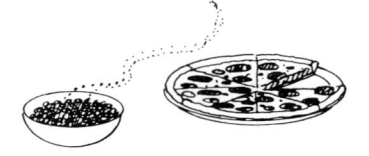

spicy foods   and condiments

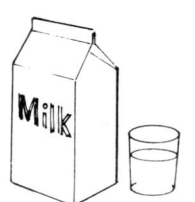

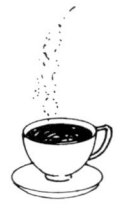

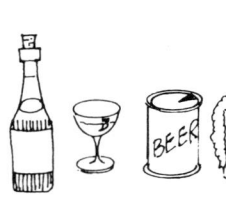

milk products   coffee   alcoholic drinks

PATIENT EDUCATION SHEET 3-6
Alopecia (Hair Loss)

Definition: Hair loss due to damage of hair cells by chemotherapy drugs (this loss is usually not permanent, and hair does grow back).

1. Get a wig or cap to use.

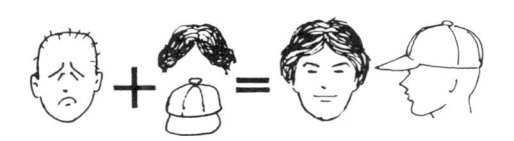

2. A hair net will be helpful to prevent lots of falling hairs.

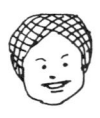

3. Avoid hair permanents or coloring.

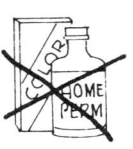

Check with your physician first.

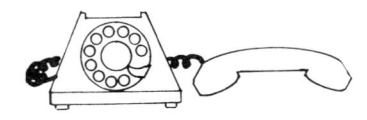

54   General Protocols

4. It is often helpful to express your feelings about your hair loss with other people . . . your doctor, your nurse, or other patients.

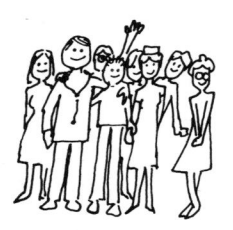

NURSING REFERENCE 3-2
Chemotherapeutic Side Effects and Drug Toxicities

Side effects/Toxicities	Drugs
Alopecia	Bleomycin sulfate (Blenoxane) Cyclophosphamide (Cytoxan) Cytosine Arabinoside (Cytosar) Dacarbazine (DTIC) Dactinomycin (Actinomycin-D) Daunomycin Hydrochloride (Duanorubicin) Doxorubicin Hydrochloride (Adriamycin) 5-Fluorouracil (5-FU) Mephalan (Alkeran) Methotrexate (Amethopterin) Nitrogen Mustard (Mustargen) Vinblastine Sulfate (Velban) Vincristine Sulfate (Oncovin)
Anaphylactic Reaction	Bleomycin (Blenoxane) Cisplatin (Cis-Platinum) Doxorubicin Hydrochloride (Adriamycin) L-Asparaginase (Asparaginase)
Cardiac Toxicity	High-dose Cyclophosamide (Cytoxan) Daunomycin Hydrochloride (Daunorubicin) Doxorubicin HCl (Adriamycin)
Cushing's Syndrome	Corticosteroids

(*continued*)

NURSING REFERENCE 3-2
(Continued)

Side effects/Toxicities	Drugs
Dermatitis, including Acne	Androgens Bleomycin Sulfate (Blenoxane) Chlorambucil (Leukeran) Cytosine Arabinoside (Ara-C, Cytosar) Daunomycin Hydrochloride (Daunorubicin) 5-Fluorouracil (5-FU) Mithramycin (Mithracin) Nitrogen Mustard (Mustargen)
Edema	Androgens Estrogens Prednisone
Feminization	Busulfan (Myleran) Estrogens
Hemorrhagic Cystitis	Cyclophosamide (Cytoxan)
Hepatotoxicity	Carmustine (BCNU) Cytosine Arabinoside (Ara-C, Cytosar) Methotrexate (Amethopterin) Mithromycin (Mithracin) 6-Mercaptopurine (6-MP) 6-Thioguanine (6-TG)

(continued)

NURSING REFERENCE 3-2
(Continued)

Side effects/Toxicities	Drugs
Hyperpigmentation	Bleomycin Sulfate (Blenoxane) Busulfan (Myleran) Carmustine (BCNU) Dactinomycin (Actinomycin-D) Doxorubicin HCl (Adriamycin) 5-Fluorouracil (5-FU)
Hypotension	Bleomycin Sulfate (Blenoxane) 5-Azacytadine (Ladakamycin) VP-16 (Etoposide)
Masculinization	Androgens Corticosteroids
Nephrotoxicity	Carmustine (BCNU) Cisplatin (Cis-Platinum) Methotrexate (Amethopterin) Mitomycin (Mitomycin C) Streptozotocin (Zanosar)
Neurotoxocity	Cisplatin (Cis-Platinum) Vinblastine Sulfate (Velban) Vincristine Sulfate (Oncovin)
Ototoxicity	Cisplatin (Cis-Platinum) High dose Cyclophasamide (Cytoxan)
Photosensitivity	5-Fluorouracil (5-FU) Methotrexate (Amethopterin)

(continued)

NURSING REFERENCE 3-2
(Continued)

Side effects/Toxicities	Drugs
Pulmonary Fibrosis	Bleomycin Sulfate (Blenoxane) Busulfan (Myleran) Carmustine (BCNU) Cyclophosamide (Cytoxan) Dacarbazine (DTIC-U) Mitomycin (Mitomycin C)
Sterility	Busulfan (Myleran) Chlorambucil (Leukeran) Cyclophosamide (Cytoxan) Methotrexate (Amethopterin) Mithramycin (Mithracin) Nitrogen Mustard (Mustargen) Thiotepa Vinblastine (Velban)

NURSING REFERENCE 3-3
Chemotherapy Delivery Systems

Purpose

Venous access systems are used when peripheral veins can no longer be used due to sclerosis or when high-dose chemotherapy needs to be infused into a major blood vessel. The peritoneal and ventricular systems are utilized to deliver chemotherapeutic agents to a specific site in larger concentrations.

Examples

- Venous Access Systems:
  - Broviac
  - Hemed
  - Hickman
  - Mediport

- Peritoneal System:
  - Tenckhoff
  - Mediport

- Ventricular System:
  - Ommaya reservoir

Teaching

- Anatomical position of catheter
- Catheter care
- Anticipated side effects
- Procurement of supplies

General Protocols

Common Problems
- Infection
- Dislodgement
- Catheter occlusion

Chapter 4
FINANCES

Anxiety
Knowledge deficit
Patient Education Sheet 4-1: Financial Resources
Nursing Reference 4-1: Medical Payment Resources
Patient Education Sheet 4-2: Financial and Legal Affairs

NURSING DIAGNOSIS

Anxiety, related to altered financial status secondary to unemployability and chronic illness

OUTCOME

Identifies resources to decrease financial stress

INTERVENTIONS

1. Determine whether client or family is aware of, or has applied for, benefits available to the client (Patient Education Sheet 4-1).
2. Determine eligibility for certain medical payment resources (Nursing Reference 4-1).
3. If client has private insurance, scrutinize policy for benefits related to payment for treatment on an inpatient as well as an outpatient basis.
4. Instruct client or family to contact loan and/or insurance office regarding possibility of disability waiver of payment of premium.
5. Encourage client and family to discuss with physician their ability to pay outstanding physician's bills.
6. Obtain referral to social worker or financial counselor.

NURSING DIAGNOSIS

Knowledge deficit, related to management of legal affairs

OUTCOME

Resolves legal affairs

INTERVENTIONS

1. Inform client and family of need to know location of all important documents (will, insurance plans, savings accounts, funeral plans, and so forth).

2. Refer client and family to appropriate people to review or discuss the following (Patient Education Sheet 4-2):

   - Will
   - Power of attorney
   - Investments
   - Insurance
   - Employee benefits
   - Gifts of property
   - Trusts
   - Guardianship

3. Refer client or family to legal aid if financially eligible.

PATIENT EDUCATION SHEET 4-1
Financial Resources

Employer

Contact personnel department of current or former employer regarding sick-leave benefits, vacation pay or time, retirement options, temporary disability insurance benefits.

Social Security Administration

Contact local Social Security Administration office regarding eligibility for total disability benefits or supplemental security income (SSI).

Veterans Administration

If eligible for veteran's benefits, contact Veteran's Administration office for possible financial assistance, even if patient is under care of a private physician or facility.

Public Welfare Office

Refer to public welfare department for medical and/or financial assistance and/or food stamps.

Housing Assistance

Contact either federal, state, or county offices regarding availability of renters' assistance (low to low-middle income and elderly eligible).

American Cancer Society

Contact local unit for possible assistance with purchase or loan of medical equipment and supplies.

Local Banking Institutions and Trust Companies

Contact bank or trust officer regarding availability of funds for particular financial problems.

Internal Revenue Service

Contact local office regarding guidelines for medical deductions, such as deduction of transportation and parking costs associated with medical care.

NURSING REFERENCE 4-1
Medical Payment Resources

Public Welfare Office

Contact or make referral to public welfare department for medical assistance.

Social Security Administration

Contact local SSA office for Medicare benefits. (Patient may qualify if he or she has been on Social Security total disability benefits for two years or is blind).

Hospitals

Contact the business/credit office regarding availability and eligibility for Hill-Burton funds or ability to write-off some expenses with endowment funds.

Veteran's Administration

If eligible for veteran's benefits, contact local Veteran's Administration office regarding care under this entitlement.

PATIENT EDUCATION SHEET 4-2
Financial and Legal Affairs

Wills

1. If a will exists:

   - Consult with lawyer regarding changes as needed.
   - Inform family members of will location, lawyer, executor of will.

2. If there is no will:

   - List all property, including the value of each item and how the title reads.
   - List all insurance policies and annuities and the beneficiaries.
   - Identify how and to whom estate is to be distributed.
   - Identify persons who may feel a right to part of estate but who are not recognized.
   - Engage a lawyer for drafting of the will. Consultation with a trust officer is also desirable if the estate valuation is greater than $50,000 and if minor children are involved.

Power of Attorney

1. A person must be mentally alert and aware of the procedures and consequences of assigning power of attorney.
2. Signing of the power of attorney must be notarized.
3. Power of attorney can be drawn up by any lawyer. It states exactly what functions are being assigned to the person assuming power of attorney.
4. Power of attorney is valid until the death of the assignee.

Savings Accounts

1. Accounts held only in one person's name will be frozen upon death.
2. Joint accounts are not frozen upon one party's death but are subject to estate taxes.

3. A lawyer or trust officer should be consulted for more detailed information.

Insurance Policies

1. Beneficiaries should be regularly updated.
2. Inform family members of policy location.

Selection of Executor

1. Selection should be made based upon the individual's knowledge of estate settlement, investment skills, and absolute trustworthiness.
2. The executor should be available when needed and willing to assume the responsibility.

Trusts

1. Living trusts are operative during one's life and avoid the necessity for publication, as in probate of a will.
2. Many types of trusts are possible. As trustee fees are usually set by state law, consultation with a trust officer to determine the type of trust and trustee is advisable.

Investments

1. Consult with broker regarding outstanding orders issued and unassigned stocks.
2. Consult with lawyer or trust officers regarding other investments.

Gifts

1. Consult with accountant regarding how and to whom gifts of property can be made.
2. Confer with lawyer or trust officer as needed.

Government Bonds

1. Purchased through a brokerage firm.
2. Can be used to pay estate taxes.

Chapter 5
GRIEF

Grieving, related to cancer diagnosis
Ineffective individual coping
Ineffective family coping
Fear
Grieving, related to impending death

NURSING DIAGNOSIS

Grieving, related to disclosure of a cancer diagnosis

OUTCOMES

Verbalizes feelings of grief
Utilizes community support groups

INTERVENTIONS

With client:

1. Arrange to have significant other present when cancer diagnosis and prognosis are being disclosed.
2. Assess client's way of coping with the impact of a cancer diagnosis.
3. Encourage client to express feeling and concerns regarding:

   - Anger and fears
   - Proposed treatment modalities
   - Multiple diagnostic studies
   - Prognosis

4. Offer to contact spiritual counselor of client's choice.
5. Inform client of availability of community support groups (example: Ostomy Club, Mastectomy Club, Make Today Count, Lost Chord Club, hospice, etc.).
6. Support client and family interaction about diagnosis, treatment, prognosis.

With family:

1. Help family understand that grieving is necessary and that each person grieves in his or her own way.

Grief 73

2. Help family members support client and each other.
3. As necessary, arrange conference between family members and involved physicians for better understanding of diagnosis, prognosis, and proposed therapy.
4. Inform family of availability of community support groups.

NURSING DIAGNOSIS

Ineffective individual coping, related to increasing deficits and protracted course of illness.

OUTCOMES

Verbalizes acceptance of increasing disability
Changes life-style as needed

INTERVENTIONS

1. Support client in coping with reality of recurrent and chronic nature of illness.
2. Reinforce physician's explanations about purpose and mode of therapies.
3. Facilitate client's identification of responsibilities that he or she is still capable of assuming.
4. Instruct client regarding:

   - Symptom management
   - Work modification

5. Encourage client to teach family members ways of doing tasks that he or she can no longer perform.
6. With client, determine leisure activities that he or she can do and that are meaningful and satisfying.

7. Involve social worker and other health professionals as appropriate regarding:

    - Counseling
    - Finances and legal affairs
    - Support system
    - Activities of daily living
    - Role reversal

8. Facilitate client's communication with significant others and family.

NURSING DIAGNOSIS

Ineffective family coping, related to increasing deficits and protracted course of illness

OUTCOMES

Verbalizes acceptance of increasing disability
Changes life-style as needed

INTERVENTIONS

1. Help family to understand client's limitations and to set realistic expectations.
2. Teach family how to assist client without detracting from his or her current ability.
3. Counsel family regarding the need to have free time and physical rest at regular intervals in order to revitalize their energies.
4. Inform family about community organizations available for respite care.
5. Assist and advise family regarding the settling of financial and legal affairs. (Encourage client's participation.)
6. Involve social worker in discussion of future plans and resources for care.

NURSING DIAGNOSIS

Fear, related to disease recurrence or treatment failure

OUTCOME

Shares fears with health professionals

INTERVENTIONS

1. Encourage verbalization of fears and/or anxieties, frustration with therapy, dissatisfaction with health care professionals.
2. Assess possible conflicts between the client's and physician's perceptions of response to treatment. Facilitate communication between the two parties.
3. Support the decision to discontinue treatment with the assurance of continued care.
4. Reassure client and family that the decision to discontinue treatment is not irrevocable.
5. Maintain a nonjudgmental attitude when the client discloses thoughts about or use of an unproven method of treatment. Provide immediate information regarding this treatment and encourage client/physician discussion.

NURSING DIAGNOSIS

Grieving, related to impending death

OUTCOME

Verbalizes feelings of grief regarding death

INTERVENTIONS

With client:

1. Assess for behavioral cues that indicate problems in dealing with impending death:

    - Anger, irritability toward family and staff
    - Frequent use of the call button
    - Inability to sleep
    - Bargaining for time
    - Loss of interest in activities of daily living (ADL), surroundings

2. Clarify what the client really fears; for example, pain, dying alone, concern for spouse, unfinished business, fear of the unknown.
3. Involve psychiatric clinical nurse specialist, social worker, spiritual counselor, hospice volunteer in helping client cope with dying process.
4. Encourage regular visits by support persons to minimize feeling of abandonment:

    - Family and friends
    - Family physician
    - Spiritual counselor
    - Hospice volunteer

Grief 79

5. Assure client that measures for symptom relief are available and will be provided.
6. Assure client that professionals are available to assist family with resolution of unfinished business and legal affairs.

With family:

1. Involve family in care of the dying client. Demonstrate how they can be helpful and comforting.
2. If the client is hospitalized, inform family daily of his or her condition.
3. Facilitate verbalization of feelings, resolution of unfinished business with client.
4. Reassure family of client's comfort by promptly providing symptomatic relief of pain, dyspnea, and nausea.
5. Inform family of imminence of client's death. Recognize that they may wish to be physically present with client at that time.
6. Inform family of availability of bereavement groups in the community.

Chapter 6
NUTRITION

Alteration in nutrition, less than body requirements, related to treatment modalities, disease process

Alteration in nutrition, less than body requirements, related to nausea and vomiting

Alteration in nutrition, less than body requirements, related to diarrhea

Alteration in nutrition, less than body requirements, related to changes in taste sensation

Alteration in nutrition, less than body requirements, related to stomatitis or esophagitis

Nursing Reference 6-1: Supplements

Patient Education Sheet 6-1: Foods Tolerated When Nauseous

Patient Education Sheet 6-2: Diarrhea Diet

Patient Education Sheet 6-3: Food Substitutions for Altered Taste Sensation

Patient Education Sheet 6-4: Bland Diet

NURSING DIAGNOSIS

Alteration in nutrition: less than body requirements, related to treatment modalities and/or disease process

OUTCOME

Identifies measures to optimize food intake

INTERVENTIONS

1. Identify external factors contributing to malnutrition:

   - Lack of socialization
   - Timing of diagnostic and therapeutic procedures
   - Preparation and appearance of food
   - Odors
   - Inability to purchase food
   - Inability to prepare own food

2. Identify internal factors contributing to malnutrition:

   - Altered taste sensation
   - Stomatitis
   - Pain
   - Depression
   - Food preferences
   - Physical deficits in the oral cavity, such as fistulas or tongue surgery

3. Institute measures to optimize food intake, such as:

   - Relief of symptoms
   - Incorporation of favorite or ethnic foods in diet
   - Scheduling of tests and therapy to minimize intrusion on meal times

Nutrition 83

- Appetite stimulants (wine or cocktail)
- Referral to community resources, such as meal delivery programs, senior citizen centers, and homemaker services

4. Teach client or family to include items from the four basic food groups daily.
5. Accurately document weight and caloric intake.
6. Monitor albumin and hemoglobin/hematocrit.
7. Seek referral to dietitian for:

   - Weight loss greater than 10 percent
   - Malabsorption problems
   - Severe symptomatology

NURSING DIAGNOSIS

Alteration in nutrition: less than body requirements, related to nausea, and/or vomiting

OUTCOME

Reports increased food intake

INTERVENTIONS

1. Determine quantity and quality of intake:

    - Total calories
    - Protein sources
    - Vitamin and mineral adequacy

2. Teach client and/or family to:

    - Make breakfast largest meal of day, with greatest amount of protein
    - Incorporate favorite, ethnic, and tolerated foods in diet (Patient Education Sheet 6-1).
    - Decrease portion size and increase frequency of meals
    - Take antiemetic or analgesic prior to meals as necessary
    - Decrease effort of eating by putting food into utensils that are easy to use and by cutting food into bite-size pieces

3. Encourage socialization during meal times and dining out

4. If appropriate, instruct client to avoid kitchen during meal preparation in order to prevent aromas from causing nausea.

5. Consult with dietitian about the use of supplements to increase quality and quantity of intake (Nursing Reference 6-1).

NURSING DIAGNOSIS

Alteration in nutrition: less than body requirements, related to diarrhea

OUTCOMES

Identifies measures to control diarrhea
Reports decrease in number of stools

INTERVENTIONS

1. Temporarily stop use of milk products and fibrous foods.
2. Obtain antidiarrheal medications. Review medications being taken for causative agent, such as antibiotics and some antacids.
3. Encourage increased intake of room-temperature liquids, fluids high in potassium and sodium.
4. Encourage use of foods that are constipating (Patient Education Sheet 6-2).
5. Explore client's previous interventions to control diarrhea. Correct misconceptions as appropriate.
6. Report presence of oily stools (steatorrhea) to physician for possible enzyme supplementation.

NURSING DIAGNOSIS

Alteration in nutrition: less than body requirements, related to changes in taste sensation

OUTCOME

Verbalizes understanding of reason for altered taste

INTERVENTIONS

1. Assess nature of taste alteration:

   - Preference for sweet or sour foods
   - Presence of bitter metallic taste
   - Loss of taste
   - Aversion to red meat
   - Increased threshold for sweet or salt

2. Explain that certain chemotherapeutic agents (Dacarbazine and Mithramycin) cause taste alterations.

3. Teach client to brush teeth and tongue or rinse mouth with a mouthwash before meals.

4. Incorporate foods that are tolerated into diet (Patient Education Sheet 6-3).

5. Caution client about food preparation if threshold for salt or sweet is increased.

NURSING DIAGNOSIS

Alteration in nutrition: less than body requirements, related to stomatitis or esophagitis

OUTCOME

Identifies measures to optimize food intake

INTERVENTIONS

1. Instruct client to apply topical anesthetics and to take analgesics prior to eating. Antacids should be given as prescribed.
2. Determine daily caloric intake.
3. Modify texture of foods, puréeing in a blender or adding gravies as necessary.
4. Encourage bland foods (Patient Education Sheet 6-4) and increased oral fluid intake.
5. Serve foods at a cooler temperature.
6. Consult with dietitian about the use of supplements to increase the quality and quantity of intake.

General Protocols

NURSING REFERENCE 6-1
Supplements

There are numerous products available for the client's use. Selection of a specific product is dependent upon client tolerance and receptivity, availability of the product in the local area, and cost. Listed below are a few of the more commonly used formulas:

I. Commercially Prepared Complete Liquid Feedings

Compleat B
Source: Meat, vegetables, milk, fruit in a feeding puréed in a blender
1,000 cc = 1,070 calories
Protein 42.8 gm, carbohydrate 128 gm, fat 42.8
Osmolality: 405 (mosm/kg of water)

Enrich
Source: Sodium and calcium caseinate, soy protein isolate, corn oil, hydrolyzed corn starch, sucrose, soy polysaceharide
1,000 cc = 1,056 calories
Protein 39.7 gm, carbohydrate 162 gm, fat 37.2 gm
Osmolality: 480 (mosm/kg of water)

Ensure
Source: Sodium and calcium caseinates, soy protein isolate, corn oil, hydrolyzed corn starch, sucrose
1,000 cc = 1,060 calories
Protein 37 gm, carbohydrate 145 gm, fat 37 gm
Osmolality 450 (mosm/kg of water)

Ensure Plus
Source: Sodium and calcium caseinates, soy protein isolate, corn oil, hydrolyzed corn starch, sucrose
1,000 cc = 1,500 calories
Protein 55 gm, carbohydrate 200 gm, fat 53 gm
Osmolality 600 (mosm/kg of water)

Isocal
Source: Calcium and sodium caseinates, soy protein isolate, soy oil, medium-chain triglycerides, maltodextrin
1,000 cc = 1,060 calories
Protein 34 gm, carbohydrate 133 gm, fat 44 gm
Osmolality 300 (mosm/kg of water)

Magnacal
Source: Sodium and calcium caseinate, partially hydrogenated soy oil, maltodextrin, sucrose
1,000 cc = 2,000 calories
Protein 70 gm, carbohydrate 250 gm, fat 80 gm
Osmolality 590 (mosm/kg of water)

Osmolite
Source: Sodium and calcium caseinate, soy protein isolate, medium-chain triglycerides, corn oil, soy oil, hydrolyzed corn starch
1,000 cc = 1,060 calories
Protein 37 gm, carbohydrate 145 gm, fat 39 gm
Osmolality 300 (mosm/kg of water)

Sustacal
Source: Calcium and sodium caseinate, soy protein isolate, partially hydrogenated soy oil, sucrose, corn syrup
1,000 cc = 1,010 calories
Protein 61 gm, carbohydrate 140 gm, fat 23 gm
Osmolality 625 (mosm/kg of water)

II. Elemental Preparations

Vital High Nitrogen
Source: Protein components (partially hydrolyzed whey and meat, and soy), free amino acids, safflower oil, medium-chain triglycerides, hydrolyzed corn starch, sucrose
1,000 cc = 1,000 calories
Protein 41.7 gm, carbohydrate 185 gm, fat 10.8 gm
Osmolality 480 (mosm/kg of water)

Vivonex
Source: Free amino acids, safflower oil, flucose oligosaccharides
1,000 cc = 1,000 calories
Protein 21 gm, carbohydrate 231 gm, fat 1.5 gm
Osmolality 550 (mosm/kg of water)

High Nitrogen Vivonex
Source: Free amino acids, safflower oil, glucose oligosaccharides
1,000 cc = 1,000 calories
Protein 44 gm, carbohydrate 210 gm, fat 0.9 gm
Osmolality 810 (mosm/kg of water)

III. Supplemental Feedings

Gevral Protein (powder)
Source: Calcium caseinate, lactose, sucrose
One-third cup powder with 200 cc water = 96 calories
Protein 15.6 gm, carbohydrate 7.1 gm, fat 0.52 gm

Instant Breakfast (powder)
Source: Nonfat dry milk, sucrose, lactose, sodium caseinate, corn syrup
One envelope powder with 240 cc milk = 291 calories
Protein 17.5 gm, carbohydrate 35 gm, fat 9 gm

Meritene
Source: Whole milk, specially processed nonfat milk, calcium caseinate, corn syrup solids, sucrose, fructose
1,000 cc = 1,000 calories
Protein 58 gm, carbohydrate 110 gm, fat 32 gm
Osmolality 505 (mosm/kg of water) (vanilla flavored)

Polycose (powder)
Source: Glucose polymers
100 gm of powder = 380 calories
Carbohydrate 94 gm
Osmolality 850 (mosm/kg of water)

Nutrition

Surgical Liquid Diet (powder)
Source: Sucrose, egg white solids, hydrolyzed corn starch, minerals
One envelope powder with 180 cc water = 140 calories
Protein 7.5 gm, carbohydrate 27.3 gm, fat 0.1 gm
Osmolality 545 (mosm/kg of water)

PATIENT EDUCATION SHEET 6-1
Foods Tolerated When Nauseous

Foods to Include

- Fat-free, clear broth
- Consommé
- Fruit drinks (Kool-Aid, Gatorade)
- Mild carbonated beverages (7-Up, gingerale)
- Clear fruit juices (apple, cranberry, grape)
- Clear, flavored gelatin
- Fortified gelatin (Vivonex, Polycose, Surgical Liquid Diet)
- Tea (hot or iced)
- Popsicle
- Soda crackers with jelly (no fat)
- Toast with jelly (no fat)

Foods to Avoid

- Overly sweet foods
- Greasy foods
- Hot or spicy foods
- Foods with strong odors
- Milk and dairy products, if not tolerated
- Coffee

PATIENT EDUCATION SHEET 6-2
Diarrhea Diet

Foods to Include

- Fat-free, clear broth
- Consommé
- Fruit drinks (Kool-Aid, Gatorade)
- Mild carbonated beverages (7-Up, gingerale). Allow beverage to lose its fizz before drinking.
- Fruit juices (apple, cranberry, guava)
- Clear, flavored gelatin
- Fortified gelatin (Vivonex, Polycose, Surgical Liquid Diet)
- Weak tea

As condition improves, the following foods may be added:

- Steamed rice
- Cream of rice
- Bananas
- Applesauce
- Mashed potatoes
- Toast with jelly (no fat)
- Crackers with jelly (no fat)

Progress to a low-roughage diet as tolerated.

Foods to Avoid

- Fatty, greasy foods
- Spicy foods

- Coffee
- Carbonated beverages containing caffeine
- Citrus juices
- Raw vegetables
- Raw fruits, except apples and bananas
- Milk and dairy products, if not tolerated

PATIENT EDUCATION SHEET 6-3
Food Substitutions for Altered Taste Sensation

Aversion to Red Meats

Substitute with:

- Poultry or fish
- Cheese and eggs
- Milk products
- Soybean products
- Legumes

Sensitivity to Sweets

Substitute with:

- Fresh or water-packed canned fruit
- Sherbets
- Salty foods

Avoid sugar substitutes.
Dilute concentrated sweets with milk or fruit juice (puddings, ice cream, sherbets).

Bitter Taste Sensation

Substitute with:

- Ice cream
- Puddings
- Lemon drops

Avoid:

- Sour foods
- Sugar substitutes
- Highly acidic foods such as tomatoes and citrus fruits

Sensitivity to Salty Foods

Avoid:

- Cured or processed meats
- High-sodium condiments such as catsup, soy sauce, Worcestershire sauce, prepared mustard, steak sauce, and so forth
- Bouillon and canned soups
- Pickles and preserved foods

PATIENT EDUCATION SHEET 6-4
Bland Diet

Purpose

The bland diet provides foods that are nonstimulating to gastric secretions. The diet must be individualized to include frequent small feedings to lower gastric acidity.

Foods to Include

- Fish, meat, and poultry (baked, broiled, roasted, steamed)
- Eggs, omelettes, souffles
- Smooth peanut butter
- Tofu (soybean cake)
- Refined and dry cereals with milk
- White bread and toast
- Rice
- Potatoes (baked, broiled, or mashed)
- Macaroni, noodles, and spaghetti
- Mild cooked vegetables such as asparagus, beets, carrots, green beans, green peas, spinach, squash
- Ripe avocados, bananas, papayas
- Canned fruit
- Fruit juices, except citrus fruits
- Plain, soft cakes and cookies (no nuts)
- Jello
- Pudding
- Custard

- Butter and margarine
- Milk and milk drinks, if tolerated

Foods to avoid

- Black pepper
- Chili powder
- Caffeine — tea, coffee, cocoa
- Alcohol

Chapter 7
ORAL CARE

Knowledge deficit
Alteration in oral mucosa
Potential for injury, gingival bleeding
Potential for injury, radiation caries
Patient Education Sheet 7-1: Tooth Brushing, Tongue Brushing, and Use of Dental Floss
Patient Education Sheet 7-2: Mouthwashes
Patient Education Sheet 7-3: Denture Care

NURSING DIAGNOSIS

Knowledge deficit, related to oral hygiene

OUTCOME

Demonstrates improved oral hygiene practices

INTERVENTIONS

1. Check client's oral cavity, being sure to assess for:

    - Large carious lesions or missing fillings
    - Loose, broken teeth or root tips
    - Inflamed, bleeding gums or food impactions
    - Coated tongue, bad breath
    - Ill-fitting dental appliances

2. Teach client and family about importance of oral care.

3. Give oral care instructions to client and/or family in the following areas:

    - Tooth and tongue brushing and use of dental floss (Patient Education Sheet 7-1)
    - Use of mouthwashes, either commercial or self-prepared solutions (Patient Education Sheet 7-2)
    - Denture care (Patient Education Sheet 7-3)

4. Recommend consultation with dentist.

5. If client has no dentist, make appropriate referral to community resources.

NURSING DIAGNOSIS

Alteration in oral mucosa, related to stomatitis

OUTCOMES

Reports decrease in pain during meal times
Practices good oral hygiene to prevent infection

INTERVENTIONS

1. Inspect mouth for changes in color, character, and continuity of mucosa:

   - Ulcers
   - Herpetic lesions
   - Infection — candida
   - Mouth tenderness
   - Pale dry mucosa

2. Mild stomatitis — mouth care is essential every 2-4 hours and before meals:

   - Rinse with mouthwash (Patient Education Sheet 7-2)
   - Brush teeth gently, avoiding trauma to mucosa
   - Floss teeth carefully, avoiding trauma to mucosa

3. Severe stomatitis — oral care is essential every 2 hours and before meals:

   - Remove dentures and do not replace
   - If tissues are too tender to brush teeth, use water pik at lowest pressure and sodium bicarbonate solution

4. Offer analgesics as prescribed by physician.

5. Explain purpose and method of using topical anesthetic. Warn client that mouth and tongue will be numb and that care must be taken to prevent biting the cheek or tongue.

NURSING DIAGNOSIS

Potential for injury, gingival bleeding, related to thrombocytopenia

OUTCOME

Uses caution in performing oral care

INTERVENTIONS

1. Monitor platelet count closely.
2. Inform physician of bleeding.
3. Teach client to:

- Rinse mouth with saline or sodium bicarbonate solutions
- Use a very soft toothbrush very gently
- Discontinue flossing

NURSING DIAGNOSIS

Potential for injury, radiation caries, related to xerostomia secondary to radiation therapy

OUTCOME

Identifies measures to prevent development of radiation caries

INTERVENTIONS

1. Assess client for dry, cracking lips and mucus-like saliva in mouth.
2. Encourage fluid intake, especially cold water, to moisten oral tissues. Recommend taking water in thermos to work.
3. Teach client to rinse mouth with saline or sodium bicarbonate solutions several times a day (Patient Education Sheet 7-2).
4. Obtain order for artificial saliva.
5. Encourage client to visit a dentist familiar with side effects of radiation therapy.
6. Reinforce dentist's explanations about need for topical application of fluoride.

PATIENT EDUCATION SHEET 7-1
Toothbrushing, Tongue Brushing, and Use of Dental Floss

Features of Preferred Toothbrush
1. Soft, rounded, multitufted bristles.
2. Even brushing plane.
3. Straight handle.
4. Small size to reach corners of mouth.

Bass Technique of Toothbrushing
1. Place bristle ends between gums and teeth and into depressions where food and plaque accumulate (Figure 14). Use short, circular strokes to remove material.

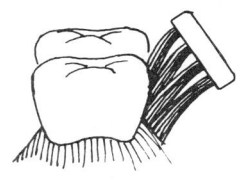

FIGURE 14

2. To clean the outside and inside surfaces of all teeth, aim the bristles of the brush at a 45-degree angle under the gums where the teeth and gums meet (Figure 15). Gently vibrate the brush back and forth in short, circular movements. This will cause the rounded nylon bristle ends to work under the gum where the bacterial plaque builds up.

FIGURE 15

3. To clean the biting surface of the teeth, vibrate the brush back and forth with short strokes so that the bristle is forced into the crevices (Figure 16).

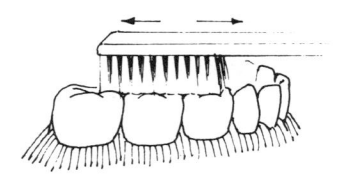

FIGURE 16

Tongue Brushing

1. With tongue extruded, hold brush handle horizontally to the middle of the tongue.

2. Place sides of brush on posterior part of tongue and lightly draw forward.

3. Rinse mouth thoroughly.

Use of Dental Floss

1. Cut an 18-inch piece of floss and wrap around fingers.

2. Place floss between each tooth and gently pull it back and forth.

3. Slide floss along tooth toward gum. Again, gently pull it back and forth.

PATIENT EDUCATION SHEET 7-2
Mouthwashes

Commercial Preparations

Dilute with water if solution causes burning sensation.

Self-prepared Solutions

Isotonic saline wash — ½ teaspoon salt added to one cup warm water

Sodium bicarbonate solution — ½ teaspoon baking soda added to one cup warm water

Half-strength peroxide solution — one part peroxide added to one part water, saline wash, or bicarbonate solution

Quarter-strength peroxide solution — one part peroxide added to three parts water, saline wash, or bicarbonate solution

PATIENT EDUCATION SHEET 7-3
Denture Care

Brushing

1. Use a soft denture brush that adapts to inner curved portion of dentures.
2. Place towel or rubber mat in sink to serve as a cushion, in case the denture should drop.
3. Grasp denture without adding squeezing pressure.
4. Hold denture low in sink.
5. Apply warm water and nonabrasive soap and brush all areas.
6. Rinse thoroughly.
7. Avoid vigorous brushing with an abrasive cleaning agent on the impression surface. This can alter fit of the denture.
8. Avoid tampering with dentures to make them fit better.

Immersions

1. Use warm water for mixing solutions and for rinsing denture. Warm water promotes action of cleaner. Avoid hot water because it can distort plastic resin.
2. Immerse dentures in plaque-reducing solution when not worn.
3. Rinse denture before placing in the mouth.

Chapter 8
PAIN

Knowledge deficit

Alteration in comfort, inadequate relief

Alteration in comfort, pain related to anxiety and fears

Ineffective individual coping

Ineffective family coping

Patient Education Sheet 8-1: Management of Side Effects

Nursing Reference 8-1: Commonly Used Narcotic Analgesics Compared with Morphine

Nursing Reference 8-2: Commonly Used Adjunctive Agents

Nursing Reference 8-3: Pain Assessment

Nursing Reference 8-4: Alternative Methods of Pain Relief

NURSING DIAGNOSIS

Knowledge deficit, related to the use of pain medications

OUTCOMES

Uses pain medications correctly
Recognizes and manages side effects

INTERVENTIONS

1. Instruct client and family about the correct use of pain medication:

   - Amount
   - Frequency
   - Route of administration

2. Clarify misconceptions about the use of analgesics:

   - Addiction
   - Tolerance
   - Overdose

3. Teach client and family how to recognize and manage side effects (Patient Education Sheet 8-1):

   - Constipation
   - Drowsiness and lethargy
   - Nausea and gastritis

4. Emphasize the importance of taking/administering the analgesic before pain becomes severe.

5. Allow the client to self-administer his or her analgesic whenever possible.

NURSING DIAGNOSIS

Alteration in comfort: pain related to inadequate relief from present prescription

OUTCOMES

Relates effective pain relief
Participates in activities of daily living

INTERVENTIONS

1. Evaluate client's behavior to verify ineffectiveness of pain medication:

    - Lack of participation in activities of daily living
    - Guarded movement or body position
    - Lack of appetite
    - Inability to sleep

2. Ask client to rate his or her pain on a scale of 1–10 (0 = no pain and 10 = unbearable pain).
3. Determine how client and family are using the prescribed analgesic. Also, review all medications, including over-the-counter drugs that are being used (Nursing Reference 8-1).
4. Assess possibility of unrelieved pain being caused by another medical condition.
5. Encourage client's use of previously successful pain-relief measures.
6. Consult with pharmacist regarding drug interactions and potentiation as necessary (Nursing Reference 8-2).
7. Communicate with physician regarding need to change pain-control regimen based upon pain assessment (Nursing Reference 8-3).

8. Reinforce physician explanation about the use of treatment modalities and special procedures to control pain (Nursing Reference 8-4).

- Chemotherapy
- Radiation therapy
- Nerve blocks—cordotomy, rhizotomy
- Intrathecal/intraventricular morphine therapy
- Continuous intravenous infusion
- Transcutaneous nerve stimulation

NURSING DIAGNOSIS

Alteration in comfort: pain related to anxiety and fears

OUTCOME

Verbalizes increase in comfort

INTERVENTIONS

1. Encourage client to verbalize fears, worries, frustrations at a time when he or she is comfortable:

   - Fear of death
   - Fear of recurrence of cancer
   - Loss of control and independence
   - Financial concerns
   - Poor support system
   - Family conflict

2. Provide information to clarify misconceptions, using language that is easily understood.
3. Facilitate communication among physician, client, and family regarding proposed medical regimen and results of diagnostic studies.
4. Administer or offer medications on a schedule agreed upon with the client.
5. Explore with client and family supportive and alternative measures for pain relief (Nursing Reference 8-4):

   - Relaxation technique
   - Rhythmical breathing patterns
   - Guided Imagery
   - Diversion

- Positioning
- Cutaneous stimulation
- Special cultural practices
- Biofeedback
- Hypnosis

6. Consult with pharmacist regarding drug combination to minimize anxiety (Nursing Reference 8-2).

7. Utilize the health teams for *pain management*:

    - Psychiatric nurse-specialist or social worker
    - Patient and family therapy
    - Recreational therapist — diversion and relaxation techniques
    - Physical therapist — positioning, program of exercises

8. Refer to pain clinic for evaluation and treatment.

NURSING DIAGNOSIS

Ineffective individual coping, related to inadequate personal resources

OUTCOMES

Verbalizes impact of pain on self
Demonstrates effective coping behaviors

INTERVENTIONS

1. Assess impact of pain upon client:

    - Fears and anxieties
    - Life-style changes

2. Increase client's sense of control by providing information about:

    - Ways to manage chronic pain
    - Cancer prognosis
    - Professional resources available

3. Identify maladaptive responses to pain:

    - Excessive alcohol consumption
    - Doctor shopping
    - Suicidal ideation

4. Refer to psychiatric clinical nurse specialist.

NURSING DIAGNOSIS

Ineffective family coping, related to client's pain

OUTCOME

Family identifies its role in alleviating pain

INTERVENTIONS

1. Assess family's responses and attitudes toward client's pain: helplessness, anger, oversolicitiousness, avoidance.
2. Evaluate impact of pain upon aspects of family's functioning:

   - Roles
   - Homelife
   - Work
   - Leisure

3. Teach family how they can support the client by:

   - Listening actively and demonstrating through their actions that they believe client has pain
   - Encouraging the use of medications as prescribed
   - Bolstering his or her confidence in the health team's ability to help with nonmedical problems
   - Maintaining contact with friends and family to prevent feelings of isolation
   - Learning and practicing, with the client, techniques to control pain

PATIENT EDUCATION SHEET 8-1
Management of Side Effects

Constipation

1. Include natural laxative and high fiber foods in diet—prunes, bran, cereals.
2. Drink lots of fluids (8 to 10 glasses a day).
3. Take stool softeners and laxatives as needed.

Drowsiness and Lethargy

1. Decrease risk of a fall by sitting on the side of bed for few minutes before standing from a lying position.
2. Prevent falls by using:

   - Cane or walker for walking
   - Rails in hallways or around the toilet
   - Side-rails on the bed
   - Night lights, hall lights

3. Avoid driving or use of hazardous equipment.
4. Avoid consumption of alcohol when feeling drowsy.

Nausea and Gastritis

1. Take pain medications with food to prevent stomach upsets.
2. Use antacid if prescribed.

NURSING REFERENCE 8-1
Commonly Used Narcotic Analgesics Compared with Morphine

Generic Name	Trade Name	Approx. Adult Dose (mg) Parenteral IM	P.O.	Duration of Action (Hours)
Morphine		10	60	3-4
Butorphanol* tartrate	Stadol	2		3-4
Codeine		130	200	3-4
Hydromorphine	Dilaudid	1.5	7.5	4
Levorphanol tartarate	Levo-Dromoran	2	4	4-5
Meperidine HCl	Demerol	75	300	2-4
Methadone HCl	Dolophine	10	20	4-5†
Oxycodone** w/APC w/actaminophen	Percodan Percocet	15	30	4
Pentazocine	Talwin	60	180	2-3
Propoxyphene HCl	Darvon Sk-65 Wygesic	240	500	3-4

Developed by: Richard Markoff, M.D., Director of Pain Treatment Center, St. Francis Hospital, Honolulu, Hawaii.
*Dosage equivalence with morphine not yet established.
**This drug is equivalent to morphine in potency and addiction liability.
†Single dose; longer in tolerant individuals.

NURSING REFERENCE 8-2
Commonly Used Adjunctive Agents

(Phenothiazines and a Comparable Nonphenothiazine)

Generic Name	Trade Name	Adult Dose Range (mg) Parenteral	P.O.	Characteristics
Phenothiazines	Thorazine	12.5–25	25–50	Antiemetic; sedative; respiratory depressive; does not potentiate analgesic effect of narcotics
Methotrimeprazine	Levoprome	10–20 q 4–6 h		Strong sedative; potentiates CNS depression of narcotics and many other drugs; analgesic; not for pediatric use
Promethazine	Phenergan	25–50	25–50	Antiemetic; sedative; antianalgesic: does not potentiate analgesic effect of narcotics
Hydroxyzine (Nonphenothiazine)	Vistaril	25–100	25 mg tid to 100 mg qid	Potentiates analgesic effect of narcotics; antiemetic; minimal respiratory depression; mildly sedative at 100mg dosage; reduces tension and anxiety

Developed by: Richard Markoff, M.D., Director of Pain Treatment Center, St. Francis Hospital, Honolulu, Hawaii.

NURSING REFERENCE 8-3
Pain Assessment

The following parameters are part of a thorough pain assessment:

Onset:

- Date of onset

Location:

- Areas where pain is present

Intensity (On a scale of 0–10, with 0 being no pain and 10 unbearable pain):

- Present pain intensity
- Worst intensity
- Least intensity

Variations:

- Usual pain pattern in 24-hour day
- Aggravating factors
- Relieving factors
- Physical/psychological symptoms that accompany pain

Treatments:

- Present medication regimen and its effects
- Previous pain medications and treatments used

Consequences:

- Effect of pain upon sleep, appetite, work, mood, etc.

- Attitudes (perception, expectations) regarding pain

Observations:

- Nonverbal expression of pain (body movements, facial expression)
- Affect

Developed by: Carolyn Wong Mau, RN, M.S.

NURSING REFERENCE 8-4
Alternative Methods of Pain Relief

Cutaneous Stimulation

Use of pressure, friction, thermal changes, chemical substances, and electrical current to stimulate nerve endings in the skin:

- Acupressure
- Massage
- Vibration
- Hot and cold applications
- Mentholated liniments
- Transcutaneous nerve stimulation

Surgical Modalities

Use of surgery to interrupt nerve pathways that transmit nerve impulses to the brain:

- Cordotomy—interruption of the lateral spinothalamic tract of the spinal cord
- Rhizotomy—transection of spinal nerve roots

Nerve Blocks

Use of chemical substances that are injected into and adjacent to the nerve to destroy nerve fibers.

Biofeedback

Use of machines that can monitor electrical currents from the body and transpose these to auditory and visual signals on one or more physiological variables. Such a process allows the client to gain control over a physiological variable.

Hypnosis

Use of self or others artificially to induce a trancelike state in which there is receptivity to suggestions and commands.

Acupuncture

Use of needles into strategic points in the body to control pain in specific areas.

Chapter 9
RADIATION THERAPY

Fears

Activity intolerance

Alteration in nutrition, less than body requirements

Alteration in skin integrity

Knowledge deficit, side effects in head and neck areas

Knowledge deficit, side effects in esophagus/chest areas

Knowledge deficit, side effects in abdominal areas

Nursing Reference 9-1: Community Resources for Transportation to Radiation Therapy

NURSING DIAGNOSIS

Fears, related to lack of knowledge about radiation treatments

OUTCOMES

Verbalizes understanding of radiation therapy
Relates reduction in pretreatment anxiety

INTERVENTIONS

1. Correct misconceptions and dispel fears client may have regarding treatment:

   - radioactivity
   - burning
   - alopecia, when the head is not the site of radiation
   - pain — "will it hurt?"

2. Reinforce radiation oncologist's explanation of how treatments shrink or kill cancer cells.

3. Orient client and family to radiation therapy department:

   - personnel
   - equipment
   - sounds emitted by machine
   - intercom system/TV monitor

4. Explain treatment procedure:

   - marking of skin
   - positioning of body, including use of lead blocks and immobilization devices
   - frequency and duration of treatments
   - being alone in the room
   - use of simulator

5. Instruct client in care of skin markings.
6. With client and family, explore housing and transportation arrangements. Consult with social worker as necessary (Nursing Reference 9-1).

NURSING DIAGNOSIS

Activity intolerance, related to fatigue induced by radiation therapy

OUTCOME

Identifies ways to conserve energy

INTERVENTIONS

1. Establish with client a daily schedule of activity, providing rest periods and spacing strenuous activities.
2. Provide assistive devices as needed — e.g., walker, wheelchair, cane.
3. Explain to family members that fatigue is real and that realistic expectations of the client must be set.
4. Consult with social worker regarding community resources available for additional support:

    - Meals on Wheels
    - Child care services
    - Chore persons
    - Church, senior volunteer assistance
    - Hospice
    - American Cancer Society — transportation

5. Advise client to schedule treatment at end of work day if working.

NURSING DIAGNOSIS

Alteration in nutrition, to less than body requirements, related to anorexia

OUTCOME

Identifies measures to optimize intake

INTERVENTIONS

1. Evaluate total caloric intake by doing a recall. Check weight regularly.
2. Instruct client and family to decrease portions of foods served and to make sure foods have eye appeal.
3. Begin supplementation if protein intake is low (Nursing Reference 6-1).
4. Encourage socialization during meals.
5. Encourage use of mouthwash prior to eating if taste is altered.
6. Teach client to take analgesic prior to eating if pain is a problem.
7. Use wine or cocktail to stimulate appetite if acceptable to client.
8. Provide rest prior to a meal and assist client with eating as needed.
9. Recommend use of foods that require little cooking. Encourage family/friends to prepare meals for client.

NURSING DIAGNOSIS

Alteration in skin integrity, related to effects of radiation

OUTCOMES

Be free of skin breakdown
Identify measures to maintain skin integrity

INTERVENTIONS

1. Explain that changes in skin color and appearance are expected.
2. Instruct client to:

   - Cleanse skin gently with mild soap and water
   - Avoid applying cosmetics, alcohol-based astringents, and mentholated lotions to radiated areas
   - Protect radiated skin from sunlight
   - Wear loose-fitting clothes and cotton underwear
   - Avoid use of adhesive tapes

3. Relieve itching of minor skin reactions (dry desquamation) with cornstarch, aquaphor, or lanolin.
4. Inspect skin folds, axillae, and perineum if these areas are included in the field of radiation.
5. Apply ointments (steroid and antibiotic) as prescribed by the physician to moist, desquamated skin.

NURSING DIAGNOSIS

Knowledge deficit, related to side effects of radiation therapy to the head and neck areas

OUTCOMES

Verbalizes understanding of side effects
Identifies measures to minimize and alleviate side effects

INTERVENTIONS

Mucositis:

1. Inspect oral mucosa for signs of mucositis

   - Color
   - Ulcerations
   - Bleeding
   - Swelling

2. Check mucosa for signs of infection

   - Whitish particles
   - Exudate
   - Odor

3. Instruct client to:

   - Rinse mouth frequently with mouthwash (Patient Education Sheet 7-2) after meals and at bedtime
   - Avoid tobacco
   - Avoid spicy foods, citrus fruits, and foods that are mechanically irritating
   - Eat room-temperature foods

Xerostomia:

1. Reinforce physician's explanation of permanent side effects of radiation treatment.

2. Instruct client to:
   - Rinse mouth frequently, especially after meals
   - Drink water whenever possible—suggest ways to have liquids accessible at work
   - Use artificial saliva as necessary
   - Lubricate lips
   - Avoid dry, bulky foods

3. Teach client to brush teeth carefully after meals (Patient Education Sheet 7-1).

Caries and Osteoradionecrosis:

1. Emphasize importance of careful oral hygiene.

2. Reinforce need to continue prophylactic treatment of teeth with fluoride gel.

3. Refer to dentist for problems with pain.

Trismus:

1. Teach client to open mouth as wide as possible, 20 times, at least three times a day.

2. Refer to dentist for mouth-opening appliance.

Alopecia:

1. Prepare client for possible permanent hair loss if more than 4,000 rads have been delivered to the head.

2. Inform client about availability of wigs and hairpieces.

3. Refer to the local units of American Cancer Society for:

- Assistance in purchase of wigs
- Counseling services regarding selection and purchase of appropriate wigs

Cerebral Edema:

1. Monitor for signs of increased intracranial pressure.
2. Inform family of need to report changes in behavior and in activities of daily living ability.

NURSING DIAGNOSIS

Knowledge deficit, related to side effects of radiation therapy to the esophagus/chest areas

OUTCOMES

Verbalizes understanding of side effects
Identifies measures for symptom management

INTERVENTIONS

Dysphagia and Esophagitis:

1. Teach client to:

    - Use topical anesthetics, antacids and/or analgesics prior to meals
    - Avoid spicy or mechanically irritating foods

2. Supplement diet if protein intake is low (Nursing Reference 6-1).

Dryness and Irritation of Trachea:

1. Encourage frequent sips of water.
2. Check with physician regarding use of humidifying respiratory treatments.
3. Teach client to take cough suppressants and/or expectorants as ordered.
4. Discourage smoking.

Radiation Pneumonitis:

1. Reinforce radiation therapist's explanation about radiation pneumonitis and symptoms to report (cough, fever, dyspnea).

2. Teach client to:

  - Use cough suppressants, especially at night
  - Humidify room air with a vaporizer
  - Increase fluid intake

NURSING DIAGNOSIS

Knowledge deficit, related to side effects of radiation therapy to the abdomen

OUTCOMES

Verbalizes understanding of side effects
Identifies measures for symptom management

INTERVENTIONS

Nausea and Vomiting:

1. Instruct client to take antiemetics as prescribed.
2. Encourage intake of foods tolerated by client (for example, soda crackers, melba toast, juices, and tea).
3. Remove noxious stimuli, such as unpleasant sights and odors (bedpans, emesis basins, urinals, dressings).

Diarrhea:

1. Monitor frequency, color, and consistency of bowel movements. Weigh client daily.
2. Teach client to:

    - Use antispasmodic or antidiarrheal medication as prescribed.
    - Increase intake of room-temperature fluids and foods low in roughage.
    - Cleanse perineal area after each bowel movement.
    - Take warm sitz baths if perineum is excoriated or hemorrhoids are painful.
    - Apply topical anesthetics as needed.

Cystitis:

1. Monitor for symptoms of urinary tract infections—frequency, urgency, pain, change in urine color, odor.
2. Encourage liberal fluid intake.
3. Teach client and family measures to cope with incontinence.
4. Stress importance of taking medications as prescribed.

NURSING REFERENCE 9-1
Community Resources for Transportation to Radiation Therapy

Careful assessment of the patient's physical condition may reveal the need for assistance with transportation arrangements. Activity constraints, driving restrictions, pain, and fatigue may make public or self-transportation to radiation treatments impossible. The following are resources commonly available in communities:

Public Welfare Office

1. Obtain physician prescription.
2. Contact public welfare office regarding transportation assistance.

American Cancer Society

1. Obtain physician prescription.
2. Contact local unit for transportation information.

Other Community Resources

1. Church groups
2. Special interest groups
3. Volunteer agencies

Chapter 10
SELF-CONCEPT

Altered self-concept related to change in or loss of a body part

Altered self-concept related to change in role performance

Nursing Reference 10-1: Counseling

NURSING DIAGNOSIS

Disturbance in self-concept, related to change in/or loss of a body part

OUTCOMES

Achieves control of bodily functions
Exhibits behaviors that demonstrate reintegration of self-concept

INTERVENTIONS

1. Demonstrate competence in caring for client.
2. Convey attitude of acceptance regarding appearance and limitations while providing care.
3. Facilitate ventilation of feelings by being alert to verbal and nonverbal cues. Provide counseling to client and family (Nursing Reference 10-1).
4. Prepare and support client and family for change in appearance.
5. Instruct and reinforce regarding methods of managing bodily functions.
6. Provide and reinforce explanations about disease and therapy so that client can make his or her own decisions about care.
7. Inform about availability of cosmetics, hairpieces, prosthetic devices, and appliances. Assist with modification and improvisations as needed.
8. Include the following in providing support:

    - Family
    - Community volunteer groups
    - Spiritual counselors

NURSING DIAGNOSIS

Disturbance in self-concept, related to change in role performance

OUTCOMES

Identifies a satisfactory role within the family
Resumes work and social activities or makes needed modifications

INTERVENTIONS

1. Identify role and responsibilities of client within his or her family.
2. Encourage client's efforts toward compensatory activities and verbalizations about the meaning of the experience.
3. Counsel family as to their expectations regarding the client's capabilities and limitations. Use reality-based examples.
4. Counsel client regarding his or her concept of self in relation to his or her family.
5. Counsel client and family regarding possibilities of:

   - New role assignments to increase or return client to a feeling of self-esteem
   - Including client in decisions affecting the family

6. Assist client with identification of self-care adaptations necessitated by return to a work schedule.
7. Explore with client physical limitations that may hinder resumption of work. Consult with physician as needed.
8. Encourage resumption of social activities.
9. Seek referral to social worker for counseling regarding vocational rehabilitation.

NURSING REFERENCE 10-1
Counseling

Definition

Process in which there is meaningful contact and interaction among nurse, patient, and family to facilitate the following:

1. Problem identification
2. Clarification of fears and misconceptions through provision of information and resource guidance
3. Minimization of stress and anxiety through development of personal and social resources and adaptive abilities

Interventions

1. Assess patient's usual methods of coping with stress.
2. Gather information on existing and anticipated problem areas.
3. Allow patient to discuss concerns by:

   - Being available to sit and talk with the patient
   - Ensuring consistency of staff assignments
   - Reflecting an attitude of relating to the patient as a person rather than to things around him or her (intravenous equipment, dressings)
   - Giving permission to let patient know it is acceptable to discuss his or her concerns

4. Focus on problems that generate dysfunctional feelings and behaviors.
5. Listen without giving false reassurances. Allow patient to ventilate fears.
6. Answer questions as honestly as possible.
7. Refer patient to appropriate health disciplines for complex specialty problems.

Chapter 11
SEXUALITY

Sexual dysfunction, related to ineffective coping

Sexual dysfunction, related to change or loss of body part

Sexual dysfunction, impotence

Sexual dysfunction, related to physical limitations

Nursing Reference 11-1: Impact of Illness and Other Treatment Modalities on the Sexuality of the Cancer Patient

NURSING DIAGNOSIS

Sexual dysfunction, related to ineffective coping

OUTCOME

Resumes usual sexual activity

INTERVENTIONS

1. Assess client's coping behaviors in dealing with his or her sexual dysfunction:

   - Denial
   - Rationalization
   - Intellectualization
   - Humor

2. Encourage client's expression of fear and concerns about diagnosis and prognosis.
3. Discuss with spouse/significant other the physical impact of illness on the client.
4. Provide information regarding alternative methods of sexual expression, community resources, and sexual therapists.

NURSING DIAGNOSIS

Sexual dysfunction, related to change or loss of a body part

OUTCOME

Resumes usual sexual activity

INTERVENTIONS

1. Assess the meaning of the change or loss of a body part for the client.
2. Assure the client that his/her feelings about fear of rejection, failure, or injury during sexual intimacy are normal. Teach the client ways to increase sexual attractiveness:

   - Wigs
   - Breast prosthesis
   - Pouch coverings
   - Personal cleanliness

3. Arrange early referral to psychiatric clinical nurse specialist and to community support groups.
4. Encourage client and spouse/significant other to share feelings regarding physical and psychological constraints to sexual intimacy.
5. Provide information regarding alternative methods of sexual expression, community resources, and sexual therapists.

NURSING DIAGNOSIS

Sexual dysfunction, related to impotence

OUTCOME

States sexual relationship is satisfactory

INTERVENTIONS

1. Listen to the client and be sensitive to cues that indicate a need to discuss his sexuality (for example, "I don't think I can be a husband to my wife any more").
2. Facilitate interaction between client and spouse/significant other about change in sexual functioning. Assure them that concern about sexuality is normal and expected.
3. Clarify misconceptions about effects of treatment on sexual performance (Nursing Reference 11-1).
4. Reinforce anatomic and physiologic reasons for possible loss of erection (Nursing Reference 11-1).
5. Inform client about the availability of penile prostheses.

NURSING DIAGNOSIS

Sexual dysfunction, related to physical limitations

OUTCOME

Identifies ways to satisfy need for sexual intimacy

INTERVENTIONS

1. Assess physical limitations to sexual relationships:

   - Pain
   - Fatigue
   - Nausea
   - Inability to assume positions
   - Dyspnea

2. Inform spouse/significant other of need to be aware of client's physical limitations.
3. Encourage open communication between client and spouse/significant other regarding sexual performance.
4. Teach techniques to enhance sexual activity

   - Rest prior to sexual intercourse
   - Use of medications to alleviate symptoms
   - Modified positions

5. Encourage client and spouse/significant other to explore mutually acceptable and satisfying expressions of sexual intimacy if intercourse is not possible.

NURSING REFERENCE 11-1
Impact of Illness and Other Treatment Modalities on the Sexuality of the Cancer Patient

Chemotherapy

General effects

- Decreased physical tolerance, varying emotional states — depression and apprehension, bodily discomforts, changes in physical appearance (alopecia, hyperpigmentation of skin, and so forth)

Specific effects (dose-related)

- Vincristine and vinblastine — Neuropathy: Possible male impotence
- Prednisone — Loss of libido
- Alkylating agents — Some drugs have potential for causing sterility: cessation of menses in female — Cytoxan; effect on spermatogenesis in male — Chlorambucil

Radiotherapy

General effects

- Same as chemotherapy

Specific effects

- Treatment fields for:
  - Testicular carcinoma — Fear of impotence (impotence usually does not occur because of dose given)
  - Rectal carcinoma and bladder carcinoma — Possible impotence (depends on treatment dose; consult with radiotherapist)

Surgery

General effects

- Decreased physical tolerance, pain, and increased anxiety level

Specific effects

- Abdominal perineal resection — Nerve damage: probable male impotence
- Total cystectomy, radical prostatectomy, and bilateral orchiectomy — Nerve damage: male impotence
- Vaginectomy and penectomy — Loss of body part
- Pelvic node dissection — Nerve damage: male impotence

Chapter 12
SUPPORT SYSTEM

Impaired home maintenance management, related to increased care needs

Impaired home maintenance management, related to tenuous support system

Impaired home maintenance management, related to care giver fatigue

Nursing Reference 12-1: Guidelines for Home Care Services

Nursing Reference 12-2: Alternative Facilities for Care

NURSING DIAGNOSIS

Impaired home maintenance management, related to increased care needs

OUTCOME

Identifies resources available to meet home care needs

INTERVENTIONS

1. Assess client's ability to function indoors (personal hygiene, dressing, preparation of meals, mobility) and outdoors (shopping, transportation, social activities).
2. Identify need for a primary care giver based on above findings.
3. Arrange for a multidisciplinary conference with primary-care person and other persons involved in care to:

   - Delineate responsibilities
   - Establish communication lines
   - Coordinate efforts
   - Set realistic expectations of client involvement
   - Identify relief persons to primary-care giver

4. Seek referral to appropriate health disciplines for comprehensive care (Nursing Reference 12-1).

NURSING DIAGNOSIS

Impaired home maintenance management, related to a tenuous support system

OUTCOMES

Identifies resources available to meet home care needs
Accepts placement in an appropriate care facility

INTERVENTIONS

1. Assess client's level of care needs.
2. Explore possibility of involving relatives and friends outside of nuclear family in care of client.
3. Arrange conference with interested persons to:

   - Discuss extent of involvement
   - Provide information regarding care required and community agencies that may furnish some assistance
   - Establish communication lines
   - Coordinate efforts

4. Utilize appropriate health disciplines (Nursing Reference 12-1).
5. Suggest services of private duty nurses if client is financially secure and such services are desired.
6. Inform client of hospice care if available.
7. Explore with client and/or family the need for placement in an appropriate care facility (Nursing Reference 12-2).

NURSING DIAGNOSIS

Impaired home maintenance management, related to fatigue of care giver

OUTCOME

Verbalizes understanding of care giver's need for respite

INTERVENTIONS

1. Encourage care giver to ventilate feelings and frustrations.
2. Help primary care giver set up a schedule that permits free time away from the client.
3. Intensify involvement of health disciplines.
4. Consider use of community resources—volunteer agencies, church groups, client sitters, hospice volunteers.
5. Initiate discussion about need for client's placement.
6. Confer with care giver's physician as needed to support care giver's health.

NURSING REFERENCE 12-1
Guidelines for Home Care Services

Home care should be considered for those clients who are unable to care for themselves because of environmental, physical, and/or psychosocial limitations and who require instruction, supervision and/or counseling, and treatment that can be met with one or more of the following services.

Nursing

1. Assessment of questionable support system at home
2. Instruction and supervision of family members in caring for the client at home
3. Provision of specific procedures and treatment:

    - Venous access care
    - Total parenteral/enteral nutrition
    - Intravenous therapy
    - Draining wound management
    - Chemotherapy administration
    - Respiratory therapy treatments
    - Ostomy care and management
    - Drawing of bloodwork

4. Emotional support and counseling on death and dying
5. Provision of home health aide services
6. Monitoring of physiological status and response to treatment

Occupational Therapy

1. Instruction in task-oriented therapeutic activities to restore or maintain physical function

2. Design, fabrication, and fitting of orthotic/self-help devices to facilitate activities of daily living
3. Assessment and modification of the physical environment as needed
4. Instruction in compensatory techniques that enhance the ability to regain independence in activities of daily living
5. Vocational and prevocational assessment; training in prevocational skills

Social Services

1. Assistance with patient's and family's financial problems
2. Assessment of patient and family support system
3. Counseling of patient and family in grief and bereavement, impact of diagnosis, body image, sexuality, settling of unfinished business, and so forth
4. Provision of emotional support to patient and family during the dying process
5. Referral of patient and family to community resources and agencies

Physical Therapy

1. Instruction and supervision of patient and family in active and passive exercises, transfer techniques, use of assistive equipment, and so forth
   - Assessment of dysfunction secondary to cancer surgery
   - Initiation of a plan to restore function
2. Integration of exercises with activities of daily living
3. Creative use of exercises to conserve patient's energy while maximizing functional return
4. Assessment and modification of physical environment to maximize safety and functioning

Nutrition

1. Instruction of patient and family in special diets
2. Counseling of patient and family on weight gain and maintenance of nutrition:

    - Assessment of reasons for anorexia
    - Fortification of diet with protein supplements
    - Initiation of use of liquid diets
    - Evaluation of caloric intake

3. Provision of consultative services to public health nurses

Dental Hygiene

1. Assessment of patient's oral hygiene
2. Instruction of patient and family in oral care
3. Initiation of comfort measures for stomatitis, xerostomia, and so forth
4. Identification of problems requiring attention of a dentist

Therapeutic Recreation

1. Assessment of activities meaningful to the patient to determine areas of high interest and motivation
2. Provision of leisure and motivational counseling to patient and family
3. Initiation of patient's recreational involvement — utilization of community resources and church groups, instruction in handicrafts, and so forth

Speech Pathology

1. Assessment and treatment of a communication disorder such as aphasia due to brain metastasis and voice problems and hearing problems due to cancer treatment
2. Instruction of patient in the use of an appliance for speech
3. Instruction of patient in esophageal speech
4. Counseling and instruction of patient and family in coping with a communication disorder

Enterostomal Therapy

1. Instruction of patient and family in ostomy and fistula management
2. Counseling regarding altered body image and functioning
3. Provision of consultative services to public health nurses

NURSING REFERENCE 12-2
Alternative Facilities for Care

Lower-Level Care Facilities

These are homes that usually provide no skilled nursing care but that may assist with the activities of daily living. They are referred to by various names in different locales — for example, care homes, adult foster homes, and rest homes. Check with the local department of health or department of social services for more specific information.

Intermediate Care Facility

This is an institution that provides skilled nursing and rehabilitation services on a periodic basis and custodial care on a routine basis. Patients in these facilities are usually those for whom there is a reduced potential for serious complications.

Skilled Nursing Facility

This is an institution that provides skilled nursing services or skilled rehabilitation services on a daily basis. These services are provided under the general direction of a physician.

Hospice

This is a place where terminally ill patients and their families can receive palliative and supportive care, with emphasis on symptom control. The focus of care is on the quality of survival instead of on the cure or the length of survival.

Part Two
SITE-SPECIFIC PROTOCOLS FOR HOSPITAL AND HOME CARE

Chapter 13
BONE CANCER

Preoperative preparation
Potential for injury
Impaired physical mobility
Alteration in comfort
Disturbance in self-concept
Nursing Reference 13-1: Leg Stump with Cast and Pylon Attachment
Patient Education Sheet 13-1: Stump Care
Nursing Reference 13-2: Phantom Limb Sensation and Pain
Nursing Reference 13-3: Stump Wrapping

PREOPERATIVE PREPARATION

Evaluation of: Muscle strength in contralateral limb and upper extremities.

Instruction about:

1. Phantom limb sensation
2. Upper extremity strengthening exercises

Introduction to:

1. Amputee
2. Prosthetist
3. Psychiatric clinical nurse specialists
4. Physical therapist

NURSING DIAGNOSIS

Potential for injury, related to hemorrhage and infection

OUTCOME

Shows evidence of stump healing

INTERVENTIONS

Hospital

Soft dressings

1. Observe for excessive bleeding. Reinforce dressings as necessary.
2. Elevate and apply ice to minimize edema in the early postoperative period.
3. Check incision line for signs of infection. Report presence of odor and persistent pain to physician.

Rigid dressings (cast with pylon attachment)

1. Keep stump level — do not elevate (Nursing Reference 13-1).
2. Check straps attached to cast to ensure that they are securely fastened (Nursing Reference 13-1).

Home

Soft dressings

1. Check incision line for healing and presence of infection.
2. Instruct client in stump care when ready for permanent prosthesis (Patient Education Sheet 13-1).

Rigid dressings (cast with pylon attachment)

1. Report to physician presence of odor from cast or persistent pain in stump.
2. Check for loosening and shrinkage of stump within cast.
3. If cast comes off, immediately apply elastic bandage to stump and notify physician.

Bone Cancer 167

NURSING DIAGNOSIS

Impaired physical mobility, related to loss of a limb

OUTCOME

Achieves early ambulation and balance

INTERVENTIONS

Hospital

1. Seek early referral to physical therapy.
2. Reinforce physical therapist's instructions regarding:

   - Upper extremity strengthening exercises
   - Gluteal and quadricep setting exercises of the unaffected leg (Patient Education Sheet 2-1)
   - Crutch walking
   - Stair climbing

3. Provide overhead trapeze.
4. Teach client the importance of lying in a prone position to prevent hip or knee flexion contracture.
5. As appropriate, reinforce explanations about the use of casting for early ambulation and stump shaping.
6. Teach client and family stump wrapping if soft dressings are used (Nursing Reference 13-3).

Home

1. Coordinate with prosthetist to ensure consistency in stump care instructions. Reinforce prosthetist's instructions about use of the stump shrinker.

2. Consult with physical therapist for continued problems with balance or gait.
3. Monitor for fatigue caused by demands of surgery, gait retraining, and chemotherapy.

NURSING DIAGNOSIS

Alteration in comfort: pain, related to phantom limb sensation or pain

OUTCOME

Relates decrease in phantom limb sensation or pain

INTERVENTIONS

Hospital

1. Ascertain occurrence of phantom limb sensation or pain. Explain that this is real (Nursing Reference 13-2).
2. Initiate measures to alleviate phantom limb sensation (Nursing Reference 13-2).
3. Consult with psychiatric clinical nurse specialist to facilitate client's coping with loss of a limb.
4. Report to physician the presence of phantom limb pain.

Home

1. Confer with appropriate health professionals if measures to alleviate phantom limb pain fail—physical therapist, occupational therapist, prosthetist, social worker, recreational therapist.
2. Seek referral to pain clinic or local rehabilitation center.

NURSING DIAGNOSIS

Disturbance in self-concept, related to loss of a limb

OUTCOME

Exhibits behaviors that demonstrate reintegration of self-concept

INTERVENTIONS

Hospital

1. Assess client and family/significant other's perceptions of loss by encouraging verbalization of feelings.
2. Support client through the grieving process by:

    - Allowing expressions of anger, denial, and depression
    - Preparing the client for the appearance of the stump during the initial dressing change
    - Encouraging participation in daily care
    - Emphasizing client's personal strengths

3. Arrange visit by amputee.
4. Counsel client and family/significant other regarding working through feelings and opening communication lines (See Self-Concept and Sexuality Protocols, Chapters 10 and 11).

Home

1. Assess status of client's coping with loss.
2. Involve the following health professionals in rehabilitating the client:

    - Prosthetist — prosthesis fitting

- Physical therapist — gait retraining
- Social worker — vocational rehabilitation

3. Suggest ways family members can help client:

- Encourage independence in activities of daily living
- Facilitate resumption of social activities

NURSING REFERENCE 13-1
Leg Stump with Cast and Pylon Attachment

1. Check straps attached to cast to ensure that they are securely fastened (Figure 17).
2. Check for extreme tightness or looseness of stump within the cast.

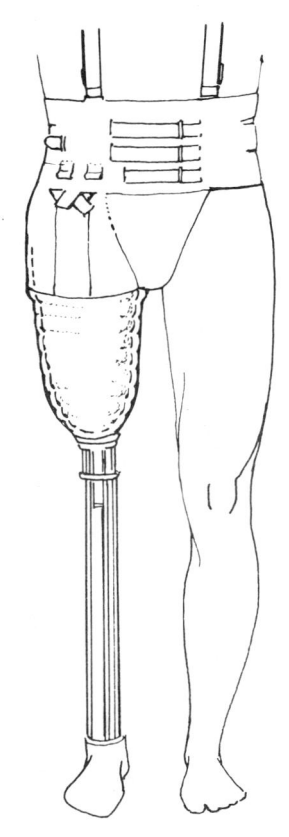

FIGURE 17

PATIENT EDUCATION SHEET 13-1
Stump Care

Purpose

To condition and maintain stump for prosthesis use

Care

Cleansing:

1. Wash stump with mild soap and water.
2. Check stump for areas of redness, blister formation, rash, calluses, and areas of pain.

Fit:

1. Check fit of stump within prosthesis. See prosthetist for shrinkage or increase in size of stump.
2. Try to maintain usual weight. Sudden rapid weight loss will result in shrinkage of stump.
3. Check prosthesis for "wear and tear."
4. See prosthetist yearly.

NURSING REFERENCE 13-2
Phantom Limb Sensation and Pain

Definitions

Phantom limb sensation is the experience of unpleasant sensations, such as itching or cramping, centered in the lost part. It occurs in the immediate postoperative period and usually fades with time. This sensation is a normal reaction to a loss of limb.

Phantom limb pain usually occurs a few weeks after surgery and resolves within a few months. On occasion, it may take years to disappear completely. Phantom pain ranges from a shooting, stabbing type of pain to continuous burning or crushing pain. Physiological causes include aberration in neural transmissions from the stump and development of neuromas on the severed nerve endings. The primary psychological cause is the patient's difficulty in resolving his or her feelings about the loss of a limb.

Interventions

Sensation:

1. Encourage ambulation.

2. Divert attention by keeping patient physically and mentally occupied.

3. Teach patient to:

 - Mentally exercise missing limb
 - Massage stump gently

Pain:

1. Report localization of pain in one particular area to physician.

2. Check with physician regarding:

 - Use of hot or cold compresses

- Medications
- Nerve block
- Acupuncture
- Transcutaneous nerve stimulation
- Hypnosis

NURSING REFERENCE 13-3

Stump Wrapping

Above-the-Knee Amputation Figure-Eight Wrapping

1. Begin with the elastic wrap at the upper thigh and proceed down and around the end of the stump (Figure 18).

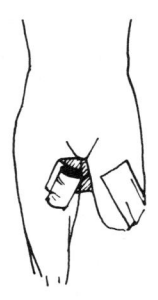

FIGURE 18

2. Continue wrapping in this spiral fashion for two more turns, carrying the wrap higher toward the groin (Figure 19).

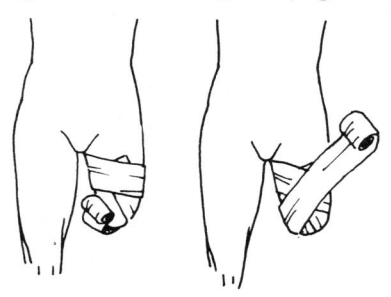

FIGURE 19

3. Begin the anchoring turn by bringing the wrap under the patient's buttocks and across the opposite hip back to the stump. (Two turns around the hip are preferred.) Secure after one last spiral turn (Figure 20).

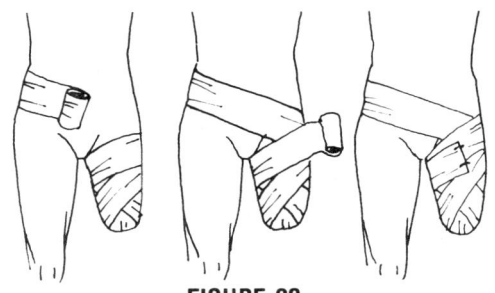

FIGURE 20

Below-the-Knee Amputation Figure-Eight Wrapping

1. Begin with elastic wrap at a point just above the knee. Proceed with a downward spiral, turn around the end of the stump, and then bring the wrap back up to the knee (figure eight) (Figure 21).

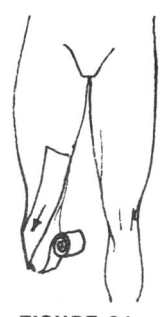

FIGURE 21

2. Continue in this figure-eight fashion for two turns (Figure 22).

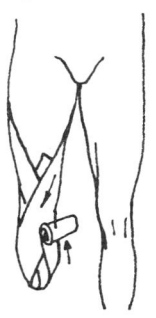

FIGURE 22

178   Site-Specific Protocols

3. Begin the anchoring turn by bringing the wrap around the thigh for only one turn and then continuing in a figure-eight fashion (Figure 23).

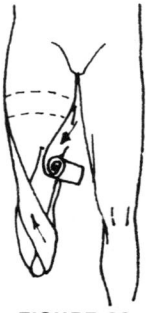

FIGURE 23

4. Secure after one last figure eight (Figure 24).

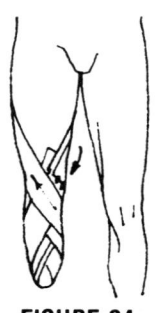

FIGURE 24

Chapter 14
BONE MARROW TRANSPLANT

Preparation of bone marrow transplant patients
Knowledge deficit, high-dose chemotherapy
Knowledge deficit, radiation
Potential for injury, infection
Alteration in nutrition, less than body requirements
Potential for injury, bleeding, related to thrombocytopenia
Activity intolerance
Potential for injury, graft versus host disease
Sensory-perceptual alteration
Ineffective individual coping
Ineffective family coping
Patient Education Sheet 14-1: Instructions to Prevent Infection
Patient Education Sheet 14-2: Reporting to the Physician
Patient Education Sheet 14-3: Bone Marrow Transplant Diet for Home Use

PREPARATION OF BONE MARROW TRANSPLANT PATIENTS

Evaluation of:

- Psychosocial status (psychiatrist)
- Family support system
- Patient's hobbies and interests
- Nutritional status
- Oral hygiene
- Life-style pattern
- Finances

Orientation to:

- Radiation therapy
- Transplant team

Instruction about:

- Bone marrow transplant procedure
- Side effects of chemotherapy and total body irradiation
- Isolation procedures and restrictions
- Placement of venous access systems

NURSING DIAGNOSIS

Knowledge deficit, related to management of side effects from high-dose chemotherapy prior to transplant

OUTCOME

Verbalizes understanding of measures to alleviate side effects

INTERVENTIONS

Hospital

1. Reinforce physician's explanations about potential side effects:

   - Nausea and vomiting
   - Alopecia
   - Stomatitis
   - Possible sterility and cardiac toxicity
   - Hemorrhagic cystitis (with high-dose Cytoxan)

2. Explain reason for:

   - Cardiac arrhythmic monitoring
   - Indwelling foley cather placement to measure urine pH and output (with high-dose Cytoxan)
   - Frequent laboratory blood studies to monitor electrolytes

3. Assure client and family of availability of:

   - Medications for symptomatic relief of nausea
   - Head coverings

NURSING DIAGNOSIS

Knowledge deficit, related to management of side effects from total body irradiation or fractionated total body irradiation prior to transplant

OUTCOME

Verbalizes understanding of measures to alleviate side effects

INTERVENTIONS

Hospital

1. Reinforce physician's explanations about potential side effects:

    - Nausea and vomiting
    - Diarrhea
    - Fever and chills
    - Parotitis and mucositis
    - Anorexia
    - Malaise
    - Skin discoloration

2. Assure client and family about availability of:

    - Medications for side effects
    - Supportive comfort measures

3. Reinforce immediacy of side effects (especially diarrhea) to client and family.
4. Reinforce physician's explanations about possibility of dry skin desquamation.
5. Reassure client and family that:

    - Total body irradiation itself will probably not cause cancer
    - The client will not be radioactive after the treatment

NURSING DIAGNOSIS

Potential for injury, related to bacterial, fungal, viral, or protozoal infection secondary to immunosuppression

OUTCOME

Be free of infection

INTERVENTIONS

Hospital

1. Provide daily shower or bath with antibacterial soap.
2. Institute oral and perineal care regimens.
3. Provide oral rinses every one to two hours if client has stomatitis (Oral Care Protocol, Chapter 7).
4. Administer antibiotics or antifungal medications as prescribed.
5. Culture body orifices and obtain specimens as indicated by protocol.
6. Recognize potential threat of septic shock with changes in vital signs.
7. Use strict aseptic technique for all intrusive procedures and for intravenous and hyperalimentation lines.
8. Inspect catheter sites, mucous membranes, and skin for signs of infection.
9. Enforce adherence to isolation procedures by all hospital personnel and family members.
10. Consult with infection control coordinator regarding environmental surveillance and infection control practices.
11. Teach client and family:

- Infection control practices needed at home (Patient Education Sheet 14-1).
- Dietary precautions and restrictions (Patient Education Sheet 14-3).

Home

1. Assess client's compliance with infection control measures.
2. Modify instructions where possible and realistic in home situation.
3. Evaluate availability and involvement of support system in encouraging client's compliance with infection control measures.
4. Assist client and family with housing arrangements when illness affects a family member.

NURSING DIAGNOSIS

Alteration in nutrition, to less than body requirements, related to side effects of chemotherapy and radiation therapy

OUTCOME

Achieves intake necessary for metabolic requirements

INTERVENTIONS

Hospital

1. Involve dietitian in evaluation and enhancement of nutritional intake.
2. Supplement intake with protein-rich milk shakes, snacks, supplements.
3. Document daily caloric intake and weight.
4. Give antiemetic and apply topical anesthetic prior to meals.
5. Administer hyperalimentation as ordered.

Home

1. Obtain baseline measurement of client's weight.
2. Determine number of calories ingested by doing a diet recall.
3. Consult with dietitian regarding the need for supplementation (Nursing Reference 6-1).

NURSING DIAGNOSIS

Potential for injury, bleeding, related to thrombocytopenia

OUTCOME

Identifies measures to decrease risk of bleeding

INTERVENTIONS

Hospital

1. Monitor coagulation profile, platelets, hemoglobin, and hematocrit as ordered by physician.
2. Observe client for symptoms of bleeding:

   - Petechiae
   - Bleeding from gums or nares or blood in urine or stool
   - Bruising
   - Headache
   - Other neurological symptoms

3. Administer washed red blood cells and irradiated blood products.
4. Use prolonged pressure on venipuncture sites.
5. Remove hazards from room — unnecessary equipment, furniture.
6. Teach client and family how to recognize symptoms of bleeding.

Home

1. Monitor platelet count, coagulation profile, hemoglobin, and hematocrit as ordered.
2. Inspect skin for signs of bleeding (petechiae and bruising).

Bone Marrow Transplant 187

3. Review and reinforce instructions regarding recognition and reporting of bleeding.

4. Review and reinforce bleeding precautions (Patient Education Sheet 3-1).

5. Assist client and family with elimination of environmental hazards.

NURSING DIAGNOSIS

Activity intolerance, related to fatigue secondary to irradiation and chemotherapy

OUTCOME

Accepts measures to conserve energy

INTERVENTIONS

Hospital

1. Restrict number of visitors and length of their visits.
2. Provide rest periods by spacing client's activities.
3. Supervise and render care with minimal demands upon client's energy stores.
4. Increase activity as tolerated.

NURSING DIAGNOSIS

Potential for injury, related to complications from graft-versus-host disease

OUTCOME

Verbalizes understanding of graft-versus-host disease

INTERVENTIONS

Hospital

1. Observe for symptoms of graft-versus-host disease in target areas:

    - Skin
    - Liver
    - Gastrointestinal tract

2. Re-explain reason for graft-versus-host disease and its prevention.
3. Be prepared to administer drugs and hyperalimentation as ordered (Methotrexate, steroids, Cytoxan, Cyclosporin A).
4. Keep accurate records of all fluid losses; especially note the character and quantity of diarrhea.
5. Relieve abdominal pain with analgesics as ordered by physician.

Home

1. Teach client/family symptoms of chronic graft-versus-host disease:

    - Skin rash, pruritis
    - Diarrhea
    - Abdominal pain

- Jaundice

2. Reinforce need for continuous, regular medical follow-up.

NURSING DIAGNOSIS

Sensory-perceptual alteration, related to prolonged confinement in protective isolation and changes in life-style patterns

OUTCOMES

Demonstrates orientation to reality
Identifies ways to minimize effect of restrictions on life-style

INTERVENTIONS

Hospital

1. Allow visits by supportive persons (family and staff).
2. Suggest client contact with peers via telephone.
3. Encourage client to share information about his hobbies and interests with nurse and to teach nurse the skills at which he or she excels.
4. Involve occupational therapist or recreational therapist in planning meaningful activities for client to perform.
5. Consult with physical therapist about a program of exercises tolerated by client.
6. Use a room with a view of the outside environment.
7. Keep client oriented to time through the appropriate use of calendar, clocks, and artificial lighting.
8. Provide radio, television, and newspapers in room.
9. Encourage family to keep client informed of events occurring at home.

Home

1. Evaluate impact of restrictions on client and family.
2. Assist client and family in the identification of ways to decrease disruptions in home life.
3. Arrange a client and family conference to discuss realistic demands on both parties.
4. Involve a social worker, as necessary, in:

   - Vocational rehabilitation
   - Role reversal
   - Schooling arrangements
   - Family counseling

NURSING DIAGNOSIS

Ineffective individual coping, related to depression in response to potentially fatal complications

OUTCOME

Verbalizes feelings of grief

INTERVENTIONS

Hospital and Home

1. Encourage verbalization of feelings regarding anguish over potential loss of life.
2. Involve family in the care of the client.
3. Consult with psychiatric clinical nurse specialist for the management of behavioral problems.
4. Confer with medical social worker and spiritual counselor as appropriate.
5. Ensure the giving of consistent information by all health team members.
6. Refer to Grief Protocol (Chapter 5).

NURSING DIAGNOSIS

Ineffective family coping, related to length of client's illness and disruption of usual life-style

OUTCOME

Identifies resources for support

INTERVENTIONS

Hospital

1. Involve psychiatric clinical nurse specialist and/or social worker in the provision of support to family members.
2. Assist family members in setting up a schedule of visits that minimizes disruption of family's daily routines.
3. Recognize symptoms of exhaustion in family members and facilitate their identification of measures to reduce it.
4. Use volunteers and friends to substitute for exhausted family members.
5. Arrange family conferences with staff for ventilation of concerns and feelings of frustration and helplessness.

Home

1. Continue family counseling with psychiatric clinical nurse and social worker.
2. Use volunteers and friends to provide transportation to various medical appointments.
3. Arrange family conferences to discuss feelings of frustration, disruptions in usual routines.

PATIENT EDUCATION SHEET 14-1
Instructions to Prevent Infection

Contact with Others

1. Avoid:

   - Contact with all persons having upper respiratory infection, infected wounds, rash
   - Contact with children under six years of age
   - Contact with children who were recently vaccinated (within five days)
   - Crowds and public gatherings
   - All animals

2. Wear a mask at home when friends visit.
3. Limit the number of friends who visit at home for approximately 100 days after discharge.
4. Check with physician regarding visiting friends in their homes.

Personal Hygiene

1. Shower daily with bactericidal soap.
2. Shampoo hair with bactericidal soap at least every other day.
3. Brush teeth after each meal. (Use soft, multitufted, even-plane toothbrush.)
4. Use own tube of toothpaste, comb, hairbrush.
5. Change clothing and underwear daily or whenever soiled.

Sexual Practices

1. Abstain from sexual intercourse (including anal and oral intercourse) for approximately 100 days or until it has been approved by the physician.

196 Site-Specific Protocols

2. May sleep in same bed as spouse so long as spouse is not infected.

Household Practices

1. Launder clothes with recommended detergent. Dry clothes in a dryer (preferred).
2. Use own set of dishes. Wash separately in hot water.
3. Vacuum cleaning preferred. (Avoid sweeping.)
4. Use of own bathroom preferred. If not possible, cleanse tub prior to bath; clean toilet if soiled before using.

Dietary Practices

1. Avoid:

   - Raw foods (fruits, vegetables, meat, fish, poultry)
   - Dairy products such as yogurt and buttermilk
   - Cold cuts
   - Restaurant or fast foods

2. Cook all meals at home.

Monitoring

1. Take temperature daily, in the afternoon. Report temperature that is two or more degrees higher than usual to physician.
2. Watch for signs of infection:

   - Colds and sore throat
   - Infected cuts

PATIENT EDUCATION SHEET 14-2
Reporting to the Physician

Call the doctor immediately for the following:

- Colds and flu
- Sore throat
- Cuts that are infected
- Fever — temperature two or more degrees higher than the usual
- Progressive rash or rash on palms, soles of feet, chest
- Diarrhea five or more times a day
- Severe abdominal pain or cramping
- A painful bruise
- Headaches that get worse and persist
- Blood in urine, stool, or sputum

PATIENT EDUCATION SHEET 14-3
Bone Marrow Transplant Diet for Home Use

Purpose

This diet eliminates foods that are carriers of psuedomonas aeruginosa and other infectious organisms and substitutes foods with a low bacteria count. Raw, uncooked foods are not allowed. Individually wrapped or contained foods are preferred.

Food Group	Foods Allowed	Foods to Avoid
I. Milk, dairy products	Fresh, whole, or skim milk, "REAL, FRESH" canned or boxed milk (any flavor), cocoa, individual canned puddings, hard cheese, ice cream, sherbet, plain popsicles, Creamsicle, Fudgsicle.	Cottage cheese, soft cheese, cream cheese, cheese spreads, sour cream, yogurt.
II. Meat or meat substitutes	Any *cooked* meat, fish, poultry. Eggs. Processed meats (reheat), dry peas, roasted nuts, peanut butter. Plain cheese pizza.	Raw eggs. Raw nuts.
III. Bread, grain	White or whole grain breads, rolls, or buns. Pancakes, waffles, french toast. Plain muffins, doughnuts, plain cereals (cooked or dry), crackers, plain potato chips, pretzels.	Cereal with dried fruit.
IV. Fruits/juice	Canned or stewed fruit. Canned fruit juices.	Fresh or fresh-frozen juices and fruit. Boxed juices. Dried fruit.

(continued)

PATIENT EDUCATION SHEET 14-3
(Continued)

Food Group	Foods Allowed	Foods to Avoid
V. Vegetables	Canned vegetable juices. Cooked fresh, frozen, or canned vegetables, pickles, olives.	All raw vegetables.
VI. Miscellaneous		
A. Fat/oils	Butter, margarine, salad dressing, sweet cream, mayonnaise, cooking oils.	None.
B. Soup	Homemade or canned, frozen or dehydrated.	None.
C. Beverage	Coffee, tea, carbonated drinks.	None.
D. Sweets	Sugar, jam, jelly, hard candy, gum, honey. Plain cookies, cake, pie, pastries, brownies.	Pastries with custard or cream fillings. Chocolate candy, chocolate chips.

Developed by: Dietary Department, Saint Francis Hospital

Chapter 15
BRAIN CANCER

Sensory-perceptual alteration, increased intracranial pressure
Impaired verbal communication
Potential for injury, seizures
Sensory-perceptual alteration, diplopia
Impaired physical mobility

NURSING DIAGNOSIS

Sensory-perceptual alteration, related to increased intracranial pressure

OUTCOMES

Verbalizes understanding of reason for behavioral changes
Identifies ways to cope with behavior changes

INTERVENTIONS

1. Monitor for mental status changes, mood fluctuations, hallucinations, and personality changes.
2. Explain reason for behavioral changes.
3. Identify and eliminate environmental hazards.
4. Teach family ways of coping with behavioral changes:

   - Change subject or activity to stop outbursts of inappropriate behavior
   - Decrease amount of stimuli
   - Make consistent demands
   - Structure daily activities

5. Refer to Support System Protocol (Chapter 12).

NURSING DIAGNOSIS

Impaired verbal communication, related to aphasia

OUTCOME

Demonstrates increased ability to communicate

INTERVENTIONS

1. Communicate in an environment free of distractions. Encourage communication at times when client is not fatigued or drowsy from medications.
2. Identify client's strongest method of communication—e.g., speech, writing, pantomime, flashcards.
3. Utilize techniques to maximize comprehension:

   - Keep conversation concrete, concise, and slow
   - Teach one concept at a time
   - Verify cognition by asking for a demonstration

4. Teach family to:

   - Assess for cues that indicate frustration in communication
   - Avoid completing sentences for the client
   - Acknowledge respectfully the client's attempts to communicate

5. Refer to speech-language pathologist as needed.

NURSING DIAGNOSIS

Potential for injury, related to seizures

OUTCOME

Verbalizes understanding of limitations imposed by seizures

INTERVENTIONS

1. Assess for increased seizure activity.
2. Explain to client reason for:

   - Taking medications regularly
   - Not driving or operating hazardous equipment
   - Eliminating alcohol consumption
   - Exercising caution while using household appliances

3. Teach family to:

   - Recognize symptoms of seizures
   - Report seizure activity patterns to the physician
   - Implement needed seizure precautions
   - Give seizure medications as prescribed
   - Eliminate environmental hazards

NURSING DIAGNOSIS

Sensory-perceptual alteration, related to diplopia

OUTCOME

Reports decrease in frustration

INTERVENTIONS

1. Explain reason for diplopia.
2. Teach client/family to:
    - Alternately patch eyes
    - Engage in activities that do not require fine work
    - Eliminate environmental hazards

NURSING DIAGNOSIS

Impaired physical mobility, related to disturbance in gait and balance

OUTCOME

Identifies ways to be safely mobile

INTERVENTIONS

1. Assess client's mobility status:

   - Gait
   - Balance
   - Stairclimbing ability
   - Endurance

2. Consult with physical therapist for appropriate assistive devices.
3. Involve client in a scheduled program of activity to increase independence, safety, and endurance.
4. Identify and eliminate environmental hazards.
5. Evaluate strengths and stressors of support system (Support System Protocol, Chapter 12).
6. Obtain referral to appropriate health team members, especially physical therapist, occupational therapist, social worker, and recreational therapist.

Chapter 16
CANCERS OF THE HEAD AND NECK

Preoperative preparation
Ineffective airway clearance
Knowledge deficit
Impaired verbal communication
Anxiety
Potential for injury, infection
Impaired physical mobility
Alteration in nutrition, less than body requirements
Disturbance in self-concept
Noncompliance
Nursing Reference 16-1: Humidification
Patient Education Sheet 16-1: Tracheostomy Care
Patient Education Sheet 16-2: Instructions for Shoulder Care
Nursing Reference 16-2: Oral Care after Head and Neck Surgery
Nursing Reference 16-3: Information on Speech Therapy Services
Nursing Reference 16-4: Types of Alaryngeal Speech

Patient Education Sheet 16-3: Payment for Purchase of Artificial Larynges and Speech Therapy Services

Patient Education Sheet 16-4: Emergency Medical Identification

Nursing Reference 16-5: Diet Instructions

Patient Education Sheet 16-5: Tracheostomy Coverings

Patient Education Sheet 16-6: Head and Neck Exercises

Nursing Reference 16-6: Deficits Caused by Head and Neck Surgery

Patient Education Sheet 16-7: Books and Pamphlets for Laryngectomy Patients

Nursing Reference 16-7: Augmentative Communication

Nursing Reference 16-8: Guidelines for Improving Clarity of Speech

Nursing Reference 16-9: Dysphagia Program

PREOPERATIVE PREPARATION

Evaluation of:

- Oral hygiene status
- Nutritional status
- Range of motion in bilateral shoulders and neck
- Possible alcohol abuse
- Communication ability
- Smoking history

Instruction about:

- Use of Intermittent Positive Pressure Breathing machine
- Alternate mode of communication

Introduction to:

- Lost Chord Club member, if having a laryngectomy
- Speech-language pathologist (Nursing Reference 16-3).

NURSING DIAGNOSIS

Ineffective airway clearance, related to the production of copious secretions secondary to the creation of tracheostomy

OUTCOME

Demonstrates increased air exchange

INTERVENTIONS

Hospital

1. Suction, utilizing aseptic technique.
2. Provide humidification and tracheostomy care (Nursing Reference 16-1).
3. Keep head of bed elevated to 30–45°.
4. Check tracheostomy ties at frequent intervals.
5. Encourage increased fluid intake as possible.
6. Obtain "neck breather" identification bracelet if tracheostomy is permanent (Patient Education Sheet 16-4).

Home

1. Assess client's method of caring for tracheostomy (Patient Education Sheet 16-1).
2. Ensure that client has a method of providing humidification of inspired air (Nursing Reference 16-1).
3. Reinforce technique as needed.
4. Ensure that client has emergency medical identification (Patient Education Sheet 16-4).

NURSING DIAGNOSIS

Knowledge deficit, related to management of tracheostomy

OUTCOME

Demonstrates ability to care for tracheostomy

INTERVENTIONS

Hospital

1. Consider barriers to learning as identified in the preoperative phase:

    - Lifelong habits—personal hygiene, smoking, compliance with medical therapy
    - Physical deficits—manual dexterity, visual/hearing deficits
    - Emotional readiness—anxiety level, acceptance
    - Availability and willingness of support person to help client

2. Initiate structured teaching plan based on strengths and limitations of client and family.

3. Review with client and family the anatomic and physiologic changes resulting from the surgical procedure:

    - Rhinnorrhea
    - Excessive secretions
    - Possible loss of taste and smell

Home

1. Review client's method of caring for tracheostomy (Patient Education Sheet 16-1).

212   Site-Specific Protocols

2. Reinforce instructions.
3. Review method of obtaining needed supplies and equipment.

Cancers of the Head and Neck

NURSING DIAGNOSIS

Impaired verbal communication, related to removal of larynx and/or structures in mouth

OUTCOME

Achieves effective method of communication

INTERVENTIONS

Hospital

1. Institute preplanned system of communication as outlined by the speech-language pathologist (Nursing Reference 16-7).
2. Support client and family as they cope with the reality of a communication deficit (Patient Education Sheet 16-7).
3. Encourage client to do oral motor exercises taught by speech-language pathologist.
4. Reinforce use of communication devices or alaryngeal speaking system (Nursing Reference 16-4).

Home

1. Observe client's method of communication.
2. Reinforce exercises and use of communication devices or system taught by speech-language pathologist (Nursing Reference 16-7).
3. Assist client with measures to improve clarity of speech (Nursing Reference 16-8).
4. Provide positive feedback for progress in achieving understandable speech.

NURSING DIAGNOSIS

Anxiety, related to fear of suffocation and inability to communicate basic needs

OUTCOME

Demonstrates behaviors that indicate decrease in anxiety

INTERVENTIONS

Hospital

1. Assess level of anxiety:

   - Frequency of calls to nurse
   - Insomnia
   - Requests/demands for family to stay at bedside

2. Respond promptly to calls for assistance. Keep promises—e.g., "I'll be right back."
3. Place client close to the nurses' station.
4. Establish system of communicating in an emergency situation.
5. Anticipate need for suctioning. Care for client in a competent, calm, and consistent manner.
6. Involve client in learning suctioning technique as early as possible.
7. Increase frequency of visits when client is being extubated and at night.

Home

1. Assess client's level of anxiety.

Cancers of the Head and Neck 215

2. Reassure client that he will not suffocate if he rolls over or pulls covers up over the tracheostomy stoma when asleep.
3. Ensure method of emergency communication with family.

NURSING DIAGNOSIS

Potential for injury, related to flap necrosis and/or infection of intraoral, neck, or facial incisions

OUTCOME

Shows evidence of wound healing

INTERVENTIONS

Hospital

1. Observe for signs of hemorrhage.
2. Suction away from intraoral suture lines.
3. Check patency of drainage catheters and amount of drainage.
4. Maintain negative pressure suction system.
5. Check circulation to flap.
6. Intraoral incision care:

    - Suction away from suture line using Yankauer tip
    - Use flashlight to inspect suture lines
    - Provide oral care frequently

7. Neck and facial incision care:

    - Gently remove crusting on suture line
    - Observe for signs of infection and necrosis

8. Flap care:

    - Check viability of flap
    - Report any signs of infection and necrosis to physician

Home

1. Evaluate client's method of caring for incisions and/or flaps.
2. Monitor for signs of wound infection or fistula formation. Report such findings to physician immediately.

NURSING DIAGNOSIS

Impaired physical mobility, related to muscle weakness secondary to resection of the sternocleidomastoid muscle and spinal accessory nerve

OUTCOME

Achieves maximum range of motion

INTERVENTIONS

Hospital

1. Teach client to squeeze rubber ball or rolled towel with affected hand.
2. Provide sling to support arm while ambulating.
3. Encourage activities of daily living with unaffected arm.
4. Explain use of affected arm to assist with activities of daily living.
5. Initiate instructions on shoulder care (Patient Education Sheet 16-2).
6. Obtain physical therapy referral from physician for head and neck exercises, shoulder strengthening, and mobility and postural alignment (Patient Education Sheet 16-3).
7. Reinforce exercises within limit of pain tolerance. Correct client when asymmetrical posture is observed.

Home

1. Measure space between scapular border and spine.
2. Report measurement to physician and seek referral for physical therapist and occupational therapist.
3. Assess for limitations in activities of daily living.

4. Instruct and reinforce about head and neck exercises (Patient Education Sheet 16-3).

NURSING DIAGNOSIS

Alteration in nutrition, to less than body requirement, related to chewing or swallowing difficulties

OUTCOME

Achieves intake necessary for metabolic requirements

INTERVENTIONS

Hospital

1. Consult with dietitian to determine:

   - Rate and volume of tube feeding
   - Calories required based on client's height and weight
   - Tolerance to specific type of formula
   - Modification in diet when oral feedings are resumed

2. Evaluate client's readiness to learn tube-feeding procedure. Teach client and/or family tube-feeding technique.

3. Encourage client independence in tube feeding.

4. Meet with physical therapist, occupational therapist, dietitian, and speech-language pathologist to facilitate resumption of oral feedings:

   - Body and head position (Nursing Reference 16-9)
   - Feeding devices
   - Food preparation and consistency (Nursing Reference 16-5)

Home

1. Assess adequacy of food intake.

Cancers of the Head and Neck 221

2. Consult with dietitian if intake is poor (Nutrition Protocol, Chapter 6).

3. Reinforce client and family instructions in program of exercises and feeding as taught by speech-language pathologist (Nursing Reference 16-9).

NURSING DIAGNOSIS

Disturbance in self-concept, related to facial and neck disfigurement and speech impediment

OUTCOME

Exhibits behaviors that demonstrate reintegration of self-concept

INTERVENTIONS

Hospital

1. Facilitate expression of feelings about:

   - Disfigurement
   - Embarrassment and rejection
   - Loss of productivity
   - Loss of sexuality

2. Avoid remarks emphasizing that noncompliant behavior resulted in extensive facial or oral surgery.
3. Respond as honestly as possible to client's questions about his or her appearance and functional abilities.
4. Arrange for Lost Chord Club volunteer to visit laryngectomy client and spouse.
5. Support client and spouse interaction.
6. Obtain early referral to speech–language pathologist, physical therapist, and psychiatric clinical nurse specialist.
7. Reinforce explanation given about reconstruction or prosthetic device.
8. Initiate discussion on the use of specific clothing and accessories to cover stoma (Patient Education Sheet 16-5).

Home

1. Assess client's acceptance of disability and disfigurement:

    - Expression of feelings
    - Participation in self-care activities
    - Participation in decision making
    - Indication of interest in resuming work
    - Use of appropriate resources for support in coping
    - Compliance with speech therapy regimen

2. Counsel significant other regarding constructive ways to support client

    - Praising clarity of speech
    - Encouraging speech therapy
    - Refraining from completing sentences or speaking for client

NURSING DIAGNOSIS

Noncompliance, related to previous health practices

OUTCOME

Exhibits behaviors that demonstrate compliance

INTERVENTIONS

Hospital

1. Assess strength of client's support system (Support System Protocol, Chapter 12).
2. Solicit client's cooperation by setting mutual goals.
3. Initiate referral to psychiatric clinical nurse specialist and appropriate community agencies
   - Home health agencies
   - Alcoholics Anonymous
   - Stop-smoking clinics

Home

1. Assess client's compliance with therapeutic regimen.
2. Reinforce need to keep medical therapy appointments.
3. Encourage participation in self-help groups: Alcoholics Anonymous, stop-smoking clinics.

NURSING REFERENCE 16-1
Humidification

Purpose

With the creation of a tracheostomy, the nasopharynx is unable to provide its vital function of humidification. An alternative method of humidification must be provided to prevent drying of the tracheal mucosa and thick, tenacious bronchial secretions.

Forms of Humidification for Postoperative Use

1. A heated nebulizer with a large bore tubing may be attached to the tracheostomy to provide humidity. This is most frequently used for continuous therapy.
2. An ultrasonic nebulizer produces a fine, cool mist of water particles; therefore a heating element is not necessary.

Forms of Humidification for Home Use

1. The steam from a bath or shower provides good humidification.
2. A portable machine for providing humidity may be used, especially at night.

PATIENT EDUCATION SHEET 16-1
Tracheostomy Care

Cleansing the Stoma

1. Wash hands with soap and water.
2. Use cotton washcloth and warm water to soften crusted mucus. Remove crust gently.
3. Lubricate skin around stoma with a thin film of water-soluble lubricant.
4. Cover stoma with cotton bib or scarf.

Bathing or Showering

1. Keep water from entering stoma with stoma shield or plastic stoma cover if showering.
2. Enclose tub by closing curtain or door. This concentrates the steam and allows the respiratory tract to be humidified.

Oral Hygiene

1. Brush teeth and tongue at least twice daily.
2. Rinse mouth often, especially after meals.

Shaving

1. Use an electric razor whenever possible.
2. When using lather, keep soap from dripping into the stoma.

Sunbathing

1. Cover stoma with bib to prevent sand or dust from entering.
2. Protect skin around neck and stoma from sunburn.

Colds

1. Avoid over-the-counter remedies for coughs, runny noses, or colds. These medications often contain ingredients that thicken and dry out mucous.
2. Use a vaporizer to thin out mucus.
3. Drink a lot of fluids.

PATIENT EDUCATION SHEET 16-2
Instructions for Shoulder Care

Posture

1. Pull back shoulders often.
2. Check posture by standing in front of mirror.
3. Sit in chair with a straight back.

Arm Support

1. Support arm in a sling when standing or walking (Figures 25 and 26 show how to apply a sling. See also Figures 43 and 44, p. 283).
2. Rest arm on cushioned support when sitting.

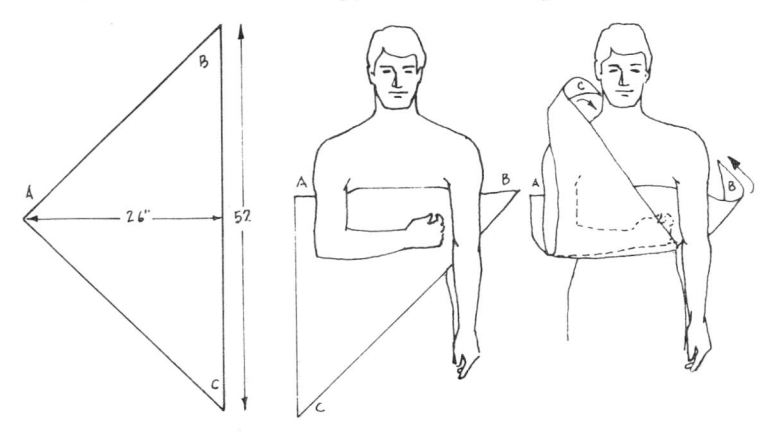

FIGURE 25

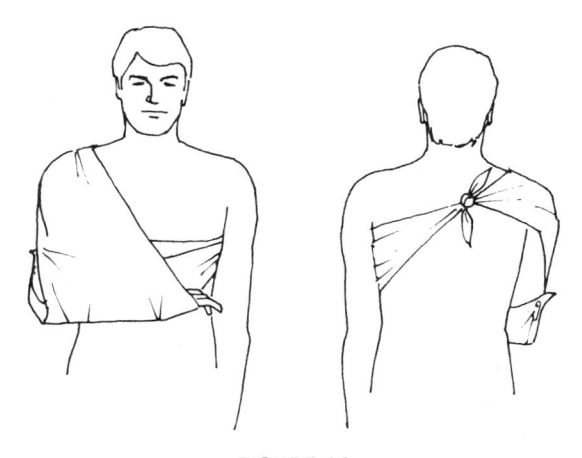

FIGURE 26

Precautions

1. Avoid carrying with the affected arm objects weighing more than two pounds.
2. Avoid lying on affected side when sleeping.

NURSING REFERENCE 16-2
Oral Care after Head and Neck Surgery

Purpose

Oral care is done, as ordered by the physician, to cleanse the oral cavity of drainage and to facilitate the healing of intraoral incisions.

Care

1. Suction using a smooth-tip Yankauer catheter. Do not suction along suture lines in mouth.
2. Use gentle stream of irrigating solution to cleanse mouth of debris. Avoid areas where the gag reflex can be stimulated.
3. When patient begins oral feedings, irrigate mouth after each meal.

NURSING REFERENCE 16-3
Information on Speech Therapy Services

1. International Association of Laryngectomees (American Cancer Society, 219 East 42nd Street, New York, New York 10017) provides free materials and gives addresses of Lost Chord Clubs in your state and facilities for speech instruction.

2. American Speech, Language, and Hearing Association (10801 Rockville Pike, Rockville, Maryland 20852) maintains a directory of speech-language pathologists.

3. Public health nurse or county health nurse can provide information on local services or can find necessary information.

4. University speech and hearing centers may have a speech and hearing clinic that can provide therapy and continued guidance.

5. Hospitals are often affiliated with a speech or hearing clinic or have speech-language pathologists of their own.

6. Local chapter staff of American Cancer Society should know what resources are available.

7. Rehabilitation centers may have speech-language pathologists.

8. State speech-language-hearing associations maintain directories of local service providers.

NURSING REFERENCE 16-4
Types of Alaryngeal Speech

Instrumental

1. *Mechanical Artificial Larynges* provide a sound that is transmitted into the oral cavity and modified by the articulators to create speech.

   - Western Electric 5C (available from Bell Telephone Company or your local telephone company). This device is held against the neck or cheek.
   - Romet Speech Aid (Romet, Box 102, 5733 Myrtle, Ridgewood, New York 11227). This device is held against the neck or cheek.
   - Aurex Neovox (844 West Adam Street, Chicago, Illinois 60602). This device is held against the neck or cheek. An intraoral adaptor is available for in-the-mouth use.
   - Servox (Siemens Corporation, 186 Wood Avenue South, Iselin, New Jersey 08830). This device is held against the neck or cheek. An intraoral adaptor is available for in-the-mouth use.
   - Cooper-Rand Speech Aid (Laminaud Company, 7670 Acacia Avenue, Mentor, Ohio 44060). This device uses an intraoral tube placed in the mouth.
   - Other instruments such as the venti voice are available. Contact your speech–language pathologist for details.

2. *Pneumatic Artificial Larynges* use lung air expired from the stoma through a tube placed in the mouth. Devices are manufactured in Denmark, Holland, and Japan. Contact your speech–language pathologist or the International Association of Laryngectomees for details.

Trachesophageal Speech

Low-resistance voice prosthesis is placed in the stoma through a surgically created esophageal fistula. Consult an eye, ear, nose, throat specialist or speech–language pathologist for details.

Esophageal Speech

Production of voice through air ejected from esophagus requires therapy from a speech-language pathologist.

PATIENT EDUCATION SHEET 16-3
Payment for Purchase of Artificial Larynges and Speech Therapy Services

Medicare—Covered under Part B

1. Obtain a prescription from the physician.
2. Send bill to Medicare if the provider does not do this.

Private Insurance—Covered under Major Medical

1. Obtain a prescription from the physician.
2. Send bill to insurance company if the provider does not do this.

Medicaid (Public Welfare Assistance)

1. Complete appropriate form for prior authorization and submit to Public Welfare Office.
2. Send approved authorization with order to provider.

PATIENT EDUCATION SHEET 16-4
Emergency Medical Identification

1. Pocket card identification: local American Cancer Society chapter
2. Bracelet or neck tag: Medic Alert Foundation, 1030 Sierra Drive, Turlock, California 95380
3. Locket (item #2403): Greeland Studios, 2403 Greeland Boulevard, Miami, Florida 33147
4. Local pharmacy
5. Local jeweler
6. Auto sticker: International Association of Laryngectomees office or civil defense office in city or state

NURSING REFERENCE 16-5
Diet Instructions

1. Nutritional problems may be associated with head and neck cancer surgery. When radical resections are done in the oropharyngeal area, there is often a long dependence on tube feedings.

   Postsurgically, if there are no complications (that is, fever, infection, and so forth), the average-sized patient generally requires 3,000 to 3,500 Kcal per day to maintain optimum nutritional status. Considerations in selecting a particular tube-feeding diet will depend on:

   - Calories required
   - Volume of formula used
   - Number of feedings in 24-hour period
   - Tolerance of patient to formula (Is patient lactose intolerant? If so, formula should not contain milk or milk products.)
   - Osmolarity of formula

2. Between-meal nourishments should be encouraged to help increase caloric and protein intake values. The use of commercial supplements, eggnogs, shakes, and so forth, is recommended.

3. The major consideration in providing the recommended diet is the individual patient's needs and tolerance. The diet should be modified in texture and consistency—whether it be bland, liquid, pureed, semisolid, or solid—to meet the patient's need.

4. Home-made preparations add variety to the diet and encourage increased appetite.

PATIENT EDUCATION SHEET 16-5
Tracheostomy Coverings

Trach Covers

- Trach covers—gauze air filters (free): American Cancer Society Chapter

- Trach covers—instructions for crocheting: New York Anamilo Club, 61 Irving Place, New York, New York 10003

- Nylon trach covers—instructions for sewing: International Association of Laryngectomees Office, 219 East 42nd Street, New York, New York 10017

Stoma Screens and Buttons

- Screen: Kenneth Lockwood, 5035 Lily Street Place, Pinellas Park, Florida 33565

- Filter base: John McClear, 61 Irving Place, New York, New York 10003

- Tube: Stoma Filter Button Company, 11100 Venice Boulevard, Culver City, California 90230

PATIENT EDUCATION SHEET 16-6
Head and Neck Exercises

Exercise

Position: Lying in bed

1. Put hands under head, elbows pointing toward ceiling (Figure 27).
2. Push elbows back into the pillow (Figure 28).
3. Repeat five times.

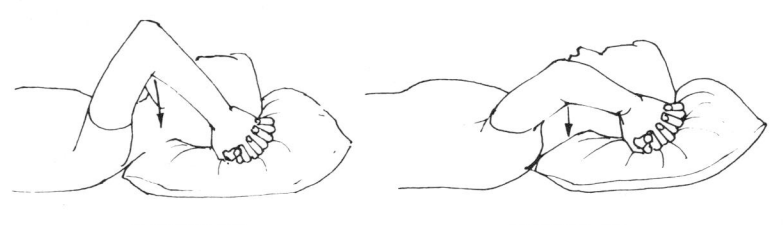

FIGURE 27   **FIGURE 28**

Exercise 2

Position: Lying in bed

1. Raise affected hand up as far as it will go, supporting elbow with the other hand as needed (Figure 29).
2. Push forward from the shoulder (Figure 30).
3. Repeat five times.

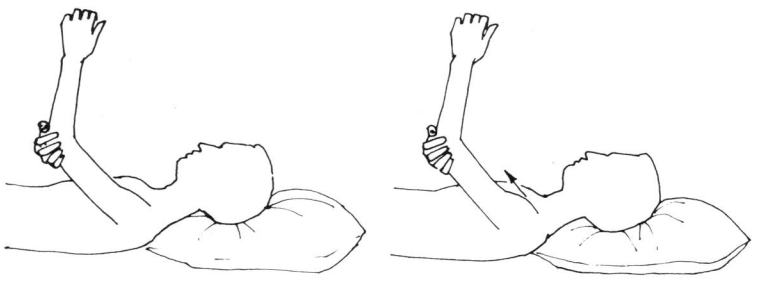

FIGURE 29   **FIGURE 30**

Cancers of the Head and Neck 239

Exercise 3

Position: Sitting with hands clasped behind the small of the back (Figure 31).

1. Inhale, bringing elbows together and pinching shoulder blades together (Figure 32).
2. Return to starting position while exhaling (Figure 33).

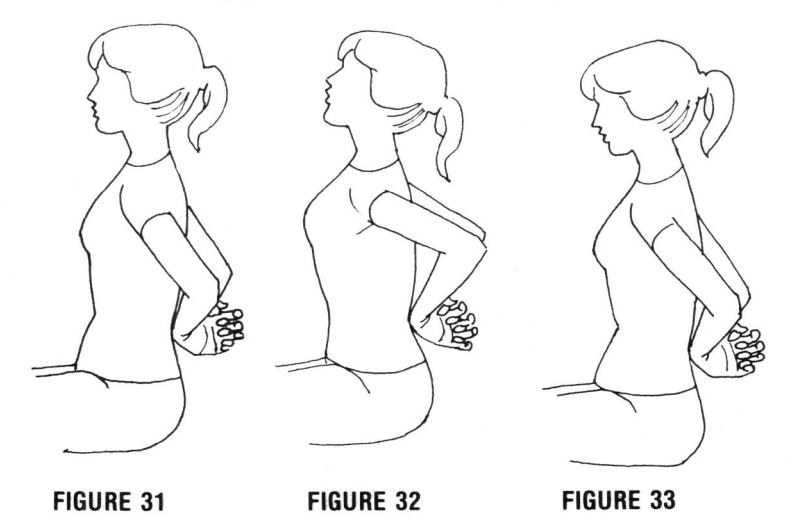

FIGURE 31 **FIGURE 32** **FIGURE 33**

NURSING REFERENCE 16-6
Deficits Caused by Head and Neck Surgery*

Procedure	Speech	Voice	Swallowing
Glossectomy	X		X
Mandibulectomy	X		X
Maxillectomy	X		X
Laryngectomy			
partial (hoarseness)		X	X
complete (loss of voice)		X	X
Radical neck dissection			
Resection of hard palate, soft palate, and/or pharyngeal wall	X	X	X
Resection of floor of mouth	X		X

*Cross reference if more than one surgical procedure is performed.

NURSING REFERENCE 16-6
(Continued)

Mastication	Taste & Smell	Facial Alteration	Neck and Shoulder Dysfunction
X	X	X	
X		X	
X		X	
	X		
	X		
			X
X	X	X	
X			

PATIENT EDUCATION SHEET 16-7
Books and Pamphlets for Laryngectomy Patients

A Handbook for the Laryngectomee, by Robert L. Keith
 Order from: The Interstate Printers and Publishers, Inc. Jackson at Van Buren, Danville, Illinois 61832.
Self-Help for the Laryngectomee, by Edmund Lauder
 Order from: Edmund Lauder, 11115 Whisper Hollow, San Antonio, Texas 78230.
Looking Forward . . . A Guidebook for the Laryngectomee
 Order from: Cancer Rehabilitation Program, Mayo Comprehensive Center, Mayo Foundation, Rochester, MN.
Your New Voice, by William Waldrop and Marie Gould
 Order from: American Cancer Society (Free).
The Laryngectomee—A Booklet for Family and Friends, by Barbara Dabul
 Order from: Interstate Printers and Publishers Inc. (order #1155), Jackson at Van Buren, Danville, Illinois 61832.

NURSING REFERENCE 16-7
Augmentative Communication

Purpose

Special devices and techniques enable the client to communicate when surgical interventions cause deficits

Devices

- Magic slate or paper and pencil
- Word/picture communication boards
- Flash cards
- Sign language
- Electronic boards
- Computers

NURSING REFERENCE 16-8
Guidelines for Improving Clarity of Speech

1. If the client is difficult to understand with an electrolarynx, the following actions are recommended:

   - Ensure that the instrument is on and that the batteries are working
   - Help the client position the appliance in the correct position on the neck or face or in the mouth
   - Remind the client to pair "voice" on and off with articulation, to extend "voice" for the length of the phrase, and to decrease the speaking rate
   - Encourage the client to rephrase or repeat unclear communication
   - Face the client while he is speaking and reduce environmental noise

2. If the client's esophageal speech is difficult to understand, the following actions are recommended:

   - Encourage the client to relax in order to reduce stoma noise and relieve head/neck tension.
   - Remind client to pair voice with articulation and to decrease the speaking rate
   - Encourage the client to rephrase or repeat unclear communication
   - Face the client while he is speaking and reduce environmental noise

NURSING REFERENCE 16-9
Dysphagia Program

Purpose

This program is designed to prevent respiratory aspiration of food and to enhance the safe passage of food through the oral, pharyngeal, and esophageal phases of swallowing.

Actions

1. Consult with speech-language pathologist to develop a plan for the proper feeding of the client.
2. Consult with dietitian to provide food of appropriate consistency.
3. Reinforce:

   - Proper placement of food in mouth
   - Head movement required to assist passage of food into pharynx
   - Importance of keeping upright for one hour after meals

4. Teach family how to feed client properly if this assistance is needed.
5. Explain why food and liquids must be kept separate.

Chapter 17
LEUKEMIA

Activity intolerance
Potential for injury, infection related to immunosuppression
Potential for injury, bleeding
Alteration in comfort, joint pain
Fear
Patient Education Sheet 17-1: Examples of Over-the-Counter Drugs Containing Aspirin and Ibuprofen

NURSING DIAGNOSIS

Activity intolerance, related to fatigue secondary to anemia

OUTCOME

Identifies ways to conserve energy

INTERVENTIONS

Hospital and Home

1. Assess degree of physical tolerance.
2. Explain reason for decreased energy level.
3. Encourage activity within limits of tolerance.
4. Help client and family determine a plan of activity that includes adequate rest periods.
5. Identify environmental barriers that can be changed or modified to decrease energy requirements.
6. Coordinate care and services by health team members.

NURSING DIAGNOSIS

Potential for injury, infection related to immunosuppression

OUTCOME

Identifies measures to reduce risk of infection

INTERVENTIONS

Hospital and Home

1. Monitor white blood cell count as ordered by physician.
2. Explain and reinforce reason for increased risk of infection.
3. Assess life-style patterns regarding hygiene and work.
4. Instruct client regarding:

    - Dental prophylaxis
    - Need for daily inspection of mouth and skin
    - Scrupulous personal hygiene
    - Avoidance of crowds and people with upper respiratory infections
    - Daily temperature monitoring (between 4:00 P.M. and 8:00 P.M.)
    - Care of cuts and wounds
    - Need to report symptoms of infection to physician immediately

5. Use strict aseptic technique when performing any procedure.

NURSING DIAGNOSIS

Potential for injury, bleeding, related to thrombocytopenia

OUTCOME

Identifies measures to minimize risk of bleeding

INTERVENTIONS

Hospital and Home

1. Monitor platelet count and coagulation profiles as ordered by physician.
2. Avoid intramuscular injections. Use the smallest gauge needle possible.
3. Explain reason for platelet counts and bleeding precautions.
4. Instruct client regarding:

   - Avoidance of aspirin and aspirin-containing products, products containing ibuprofen (Patient Education Sheet 17-1).
   - Use of prolonged pressure on venipuncture sites and bruises.
   - Use of an electric razor for shaving.
   - Possibility of menstrual cycle irregularities in women.
   - Need to inspect mouth, skin, stool, and urine for signs of bleeding.
   - Reporting of persistent, progressive headache to physician immediately.
   - Need to curtail strenuous physical activities
   - Use of stool softener

5. Assist client with planning and modifying activities in a way he or she can accept.
6. If client has bled and formed a clot, instruct client that it must not be removed.

Leukemia 251

NURSING DIAGNOSIS

Alteration in comfort: pain in joints, related to hyperuricemia

OUTCOME

Expresses pain relief or increased comfort

INTERVENTIONS

Hospital and Home

1. Monitor serum uric acid as ordered by physician.
2. Encourage increased fluid intake.
3. Reinforce reason for taking uricosuric drugs as a prophylactic basis.
4. Teach client and family about avoiding high purine foods (Patient Education Sheet 3-2).

NURSING DIAGNOSIS

Fear, related to exacerbation of leukemia

OUTCOME

Shares fears with health professionals and support groups

INTERVENTIONS

Hospital and Home

1. Interact with client and family members to answer questions, clarify misconceptions, and allay fears.
2. Reinforce physician's explanations about proposed chemotherapy.
3. Encourage rooming-in by family members.
4. Involve spiritual counselor if client so desires.
5. Involve community and church support groups — Candlelighters, Make Today Count, Hospice, American Cancer Society, bereavement groups.

PATIENT EDUCATION SHEET 17-1
Examples of Over-the-Counter Drugs Containing Aspirin and Ibuprofen

Aspirin

- Alka-Seltzer
- Anacin
- A.P.C.
- A.S.A. Compound
- Ascriptin
- Bufferin
- Cope
- Coricidin
- Dristan
- Ecotrin
- Empirin Compound
- Excedrin
- Measurin
- Midol
- P-A-C
- Vanquish

Ibuprofen

- Advil
- Nuprin
- Rufen

NURSING DIAGNOSIS

Impaired gas exchange, related to surgical entry into pleural space and/or atelectasis

OUTCOME

Achieves maximum ventilation and aeration of lungs

INTERVENTIONS

Hospital

1. Maintain underwater seal drainage and proper functioning of equipment (Nursing Reference 18-2).
2. Auscultate lungs.
3. Assess contributing factors such as:

   - Pain
   - Inactivity
   - Improper breathing techniques
   - Anxiety

4. Encourage breathing techniques to facilitate gas exchange:

   - Staccato coughing
   - Use of incentive spirometer
   - Chest physiotherapy (Nursing Reference 18-1)

5. Encourage progressive ambulation.
6. Give pain medication prior to treatments and activity.

Site-Specific Protocols

Home

1. Auscultate lungs each visit.
2. Reinforce or initiate exercises in pursed-lip and abdominal breathing (Patient Education Sheet 18-1).
3. Obtain order for chest physiotherapy and respiratory appliances as needed (Nursing Reference 18-1).
4. Teach chest physiotherapy to family members.

NURSING DIAGNOSIS

Ineffective airway clearance, related to viscosity of secretions

OUTCOME

Demonstrates increased air exchange

INTERVENTIONS

Hospital

1. Auscultate lungs.
2. Encourage stir-up exercises:

    - Frequent position changes
    - Progressive ambulation
    - Deep breathing and coughing
    - Wiggling toes and opening/closing fingers

3. Provide optimal fluid intake.
4. Confer with respiratory therapist regarding appropriate respiratory treatments.
5. Discuss factors that increase the amount of viscosity of mucus:

    - Cigarette smoking
    - Poor fluid intake
    - OTC drugs like antihistamines
    - Colds
    - Environmental pollutants—smog, pollens, molds, etc.

Home

1. Assess respiratory status.
2. Reinforce instructions about clearing secretions and dealing with viscous mucus.
3. Encourage client to seek flu/pneumonia immunization.

NURSING DIAGNOSIS

Impaired physical mobility (shoulder), related to pain of surgical incision

OUTCOME

Attains maximum shoulder range of motion and posture

INTERVENTIONS

Hospital

1. Position arm functionally.
2. Administer pain medications.
3. Perform passive range-of-motion exercises.
4. Initiate instruction in active-assisted and active exercises (Patient Education Sheet 18-2).
5. Obtain physical therapist or occupational therapist referral if client had prior limitations in range of motion.

Home

1. Obtain baseline measurement of range of motion in affected shoulder.
2. Reinforce or instruct in shoulder active range-of-motion exercises (Patient Education Sheet 18-2).
3. Obtain referral for occupational therapist or physical therapist if dysfunction persists.

NURSING DIAGNOSIS

Activity intolerance, related to dyspnea secondary to limited lung reserve or disease progression

OUTCOME

Performs activities within limits of physical tolerance

INTERVENTIONS

Hospital

1. Mutually establish goals for graded exercises.
2. Teach client to use breathing patterns while doing exercises and activities such as stair climbing.
3. Instruct client in energy conservation techniques:

    - Spacing activities with rest periods
    - Selecting foods that are easily chewed

4. Report to physician symptoms suggesting the need for supplemental oxygen.

Home

1. Reinforce or instruct in ways to conserve energy while doing daily activities.
2. Consult with occupational therapist for work simplification.
3. Evaluate need for supplemental oxygen.

PATIENT EDUCATION SHEET 18-1
Pursed-Lip and Abdominal Breathing Exercise

Position: Reclining

1. Concentrate on breathing with the abdomen.
2. Exhale slowly through pursed lips (Figure 34), contracting the abdominal muscles (Figure 35).

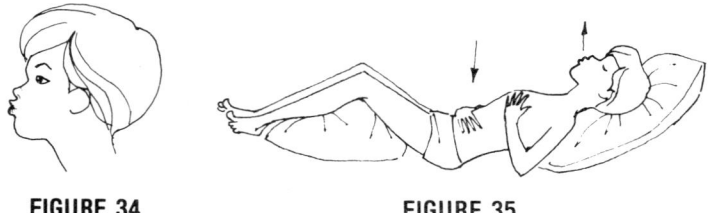

FIGURE 34   **FIGURE 35**

3. Keep the upper thorax relaxed and free of movement.
4. Relax the abdominal muscles and push them up, inhaling through the nose (Figure 36).

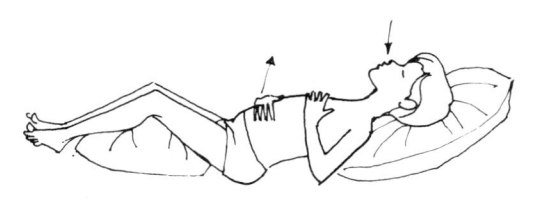

FIGURE 36

5. Always start exercise with exhalation and empty the lungs completely. Inhalation will come naturally.

After mastering the exercises in the reclining position, practice in a sitting position.

NURSING REFERENCE 18-1
Chest Percussion

1. Tap chest wall with cupped hands (Figure 37) over area of lung to be drained. (Cupped hands form air pockets that produce a hollow sound when properly done.)

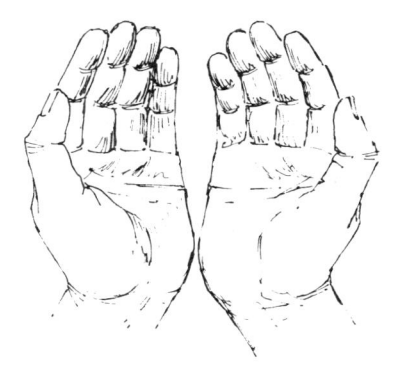

FIGURE 37

2. Use both hands alternately, keeping arm and wrist relaxed (Figure 38).

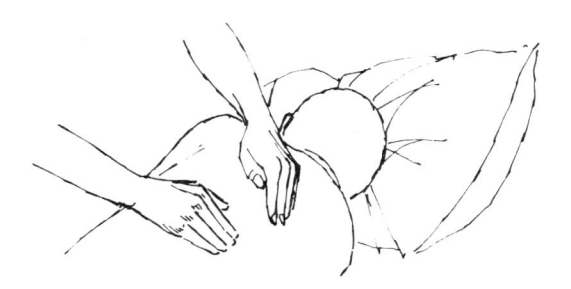

FIGURE 38

3. Percuss for at least one minute over each area of the lung involved.

PATIENT EDUCATION SHEET 18-2
Post-Thoracotomy Exercises

Exercise 1

Position: Sitting with arms extended in front of you, elbows straight (Figure 39).

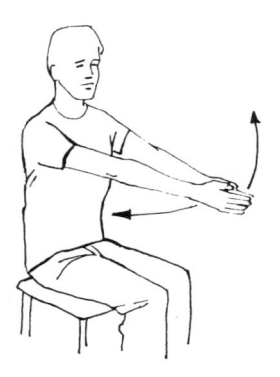

FIGURE 39

1. While inhaling, spread arms apart slowly, palms facing up. Continue to spread arms until you feel you are pinching your shoulder blades together (Figure 40).
2. While exhaling, return to your starting position.

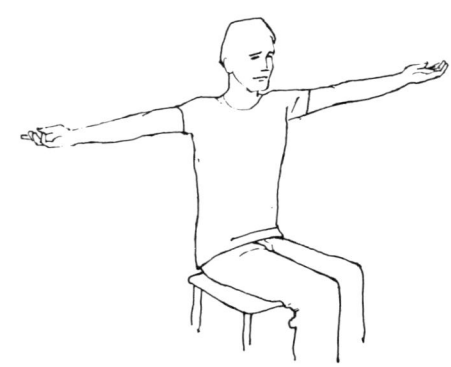

FIGURE 40

Exercise 2

Position: Sitting with elbows straight and hands clasped on lap (Figure 41).

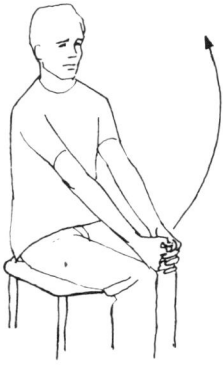

FIGURE 41

1. Raise both hands up toward your head as far as possible, inhaling slowly (Figure 42).

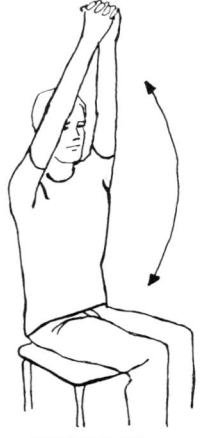

FIGURE 42

2. Lower arms to starting position, while exhaling.

NURSING REFERENCE 18-2
Care of Chest Tubes

1. Check that all connections are airtight and securely taped.
2. Ensure that tubing is not kinked. Kinked tubing may cause a tension pneumothorax.
3. Note character and amount of drainage. Correlate amount of drainage with vital signs. Notify physician immediately if drainage exceeds 100 cc in one hour.
4. Bubbling in the underwater seal bottle indicates air is being expelled from the intrapleural space. Late bubbling may indicate a bronchopleural fistula, a tear in the lung, or a leak in the wound site. Never clamp a bubbling chest tube. This can cause a tension pneumothorax and a fatal mediastinal shift. If the underwater seal bottle breaks in a patient with a bubbling chest tube, leave the tube unclamped and place it in an available container under water.
5. Milk tubing periodically from patient's chest tube toward the drainage bottle.
6. Note fluctuation of fluid in the tubing. Cessation of fluid fluctuation indicates reexpansion of the lung.

Chapter 19
BREAST CANCER

Preoperative preparation
Potential for injury, serous fluid collection
Potential for injury, wound infection
Potential fluid volume excess, lymphedema
Impaired physical mobility
Disturbance in self-concept
Anxiety
Knowledge deficit
Patient Education Sheet 19-1: The Jackson-Pratt Drain
Patient Education Sheet 19-2: Arm Support
Nursing Reference 19-1: Arm Circumference Measurement
Patient Education Sheet 19-3: Postoperative Exercises
Nursing Reference 19-2: Mastectomy Exercises
Patient Education Sheet 19-4: Post-Mastectomy Exercises
Patient Education Sheet 19-5: Suggestions for Preventing Infection and Swelling of Affected Arm and Hand
Patient Education Sheet 19-6: Postural Exercise

Patient Education Sheet 19-7: Activity Guidelines for Mastectomy Patients

Patient Education Sheet 19-8: Temporary Prosthesis

Patient Education Sheet 19-9: Permanent Prosthesis Information

Nursing Reference 19-3: Self-Help Programs

PREOPERATIVE PREPARATION

Evaluation of:

- Range of motion in bilateral arms and shoulders
- Posture

Baseline measurements of:

- Arm circumference 7 cm above the olecranon and 11 cm below the olecranon

Assessment of knowledge regarding:

- Treatment options
- Breast reconstruction

NURSING DIAGNOSIS

Potential for injury, related to collection of serous fluid under flap

OUTCOME

Achieves wound healing

INTERVENTIONS

Hospital

1. Immediately after surgery, check wound for:

   - Color
   - Signs of swelling
   - Hematoma formation

2. Ensure that drains are intact and/or that drainage catheters are functioning properly (Patient Education Sheet 19-1).

3. Initiate instructions on the care of Jackson Pratt suction device if client is to be discharged with drains in place.

Home

1. Check if drains are intact and draining properly.

2. Reinforce instructions:

   - Accurate measurement of drainage
   - Compression of Jackson Pratt bulb

NURSING DIAGNOSIS

Potential for injury, related to wound infection

OUTCOME

Shows no evidence of wound infection

INTERVENTIONS

Hospital

1. Use strict aseptic technique when changing dressing.
2. Instruct client to avoid touching wound, particularly when it is exposed.
3. Initiate instructions on wound care.
4. Explain usual postoperative problems associated with wound healing:

   - Tightness
   - Numbness, tingling sensation in chest and under arm pits

Home

1. Assess client's method of wound care.
2. Check incision for signs of infection — redness, swelling, tenderness, purulent discharge.
3. If wound becomes infected, assist or instruct client in care as ordered by physician.
4. Instruct regarding need for compliance with antibiotic therapy.

NURSING DIAGNOSIS

Potential fluid volume excess, related to lymphedema secondary to axillary node dissection

OUTCOME

Exhibits minimal lymphedema of arm

INTERVENTIONS

Hospital

1. Elevate arm while in bed to promote gravity drainage of lymph fluid.
2. Provide arm sling or cushioned support for use when ambulating (Patient Education Sheet 19-2).
3. Place sign reminding hospital personnel not to use affected arm for blood-pressure readings, intravenous procedures, blood work, or injections.
4. Encourage use of arm for simple activities of daily living, such as reaching for glass, combing hair, and brushing teeth.
5. Apply elastic sleeve or elastic bandages as ordered.
6. Measure and record arm circumference above and below elbow daily (Nursing Reference 19-1).
7. Begin program of exercises with physician's approval (Nursing Reference 19-2 and Patient Education Sheet 19-4).
8. Instruct client about hand and arm care (Patient Education Sheet 19-5).

Home

1. Obtain baseline measurement of arm circumferences above and below elbow (Nursing Reference 19-1). Then measure arm circumference weekly. Report increases greater than 3 cm to physician.

2. Review instructions about the prevention of infection and swelling (Patient Education Sheet 19-5).

3. Encourage continued use of arm in activities of daily living.

NURSING DIAGNOSIS

Impaired physical mobility, related to limited range of motion and shoulder imbalance

OUTCOMES

Demonstrates exercises to attain maximum strength and range of motion
Integrates exercises into activities of daily living

INTERVENTIONS

Hospital

1. Teach postoperative exercises (Patient Education Sheet 19-3).

2. Encourage use of affected arm in self care—brushing teeth, brushing hair, and bathing.

3. Identify fears that contribute to immobility of the affected arm—injuring incision and pain.

4. Begin program of active exercises (Nursing Reference 19-2 and Patient Education Sheet 19-4). Exercises may be delayed with a skin graft.

5. Teach postural exercises (Patient Education Sheet 19-6).

6. Review instructions for continuing and increasing activity after discharge (Patient Education Sheet 19-7).

Home

1. Assess the type and frequency of exercises performed.

2. Check for arm heaviness and shoulder stiffness.

3. Instruct regarding exercises as necessary (Nursing Reference 19-2 and Patient Education Sheets 19-4 and 19-5).

4. Encourage gradual increase in use of affected arm for household chores.

5. Discuss use of temporary prosthesis to improve posture.

NURSING DIAGNOSIS

Disturbance in self-concept, related to loss of breast and disfiguring scar.

OUTCOME

Demonstrates behaviors that indicate reintegration of self-concept

INTERVENTIONS

Hospital

1. Encourage verbalization of feelings by being alert for verbal and nonverbal cues.
2. Support client's interaction with spouse or significant other.
3. Prepare client for appearance of the incision.
4. Arrange visit by an American Cancer Society's Reach to Recovery volunteer (Nursing Reference 19-3).
5. Provide information about Encore Program (Nursing Reference 19-3).
6. Instruct client regarding use of temporary and permanent prosthesis (Patient Education Sheets 19-8 and 19-9).
7. Explore option of breast reconstruction if client indicates interest.
8. Provide client with book, *First You Cry*, by Betty Rollins.

Home

1. Facilitate grieving process by:

    - Actively listening to client's fears and feelings of anger, guilt, hopelessness

- Allowing client to clarify concerns about the mastectomy scar

2. Refer to support groups—Reach to Recovery group, Encore program.

3. Assist client in fabricating and using a temporary prosthesis (Patient Education Sheet 19-8).

4. Provide and review information on prosthesis and where it can be purchased.

5. Explore option of breast reconstruction if client indicates interest.

NURSING DIAGNOSIS

Anxiety, related to misconceptions and uncertainty about proposed therapy and future

OUTCOME

Demonstrates behaviors that indicate decrease in level of anxiety

INTERVENTIONS

Hospital and Home

1. Clarify misconceptions, involving physician, other health team member, and Reach to Recovery volunteer as appropriate.
2. Prepare client for possible adjuvant chemotherapy or radiation.
3. Review informational brochures with client and family. Respond to questions honestly and in an unbiased way.
4. Avoid oversimplifying treatment options to minimize client fears.
5. Encourage client to discuss with physician her concerns about the type of therapy proposed, media information, and well-meaning advice from friends and family.
6. Support client's decision for second opinion.
7. Acknowledge client preoccupation with the future by encouraging discussion about cancer recurrence and death.

NURSING DIAGNOSIS

Knowledge deficit, related to risk of cancer in contralateral breast and in female blood relatives

OUTCOME

Performs monthly breast self-examination

INTERVENTIONS

Hospital and Home

1. Teach and review with client how to do a breast self-examination.
2. Teach available and interested family members about self-examination and their increased risk of breast cancer.

PATIENT EDUCATION SHEET 19-1
The Jackson-Pratt Drain

Purpose

Provide drainage of wound exudate, promoting wound healing and flap adherence to chest wall

Steps

1. Wash hands with soap and water.
2. Open emptying port cap. Pour out contents into a container and set aside. Wipe port with alcohol.
3. Gently squeeze the bulb until it is flattened. Recap the port. (If the bulb inflates quickly, it usually indicates a leak in the system that should be brought to the physician's attention.)
4. Resecure device to clothing.
5. Measure amount of fluid removed from the bulb and record it.
6. Empty fluid into toilet. Wash container and hands thoroughly.

PATIENT EDUCATION SHEET 19-2
Arm Support

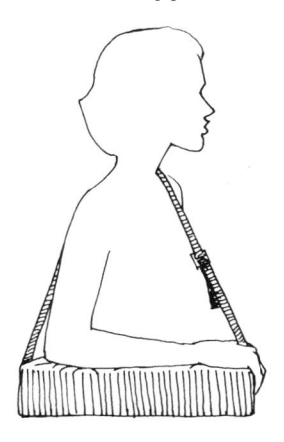

FIGURE 43. CUSHION. (SEE ALSO FIGURES 25 AND 26, PP. 228–229)

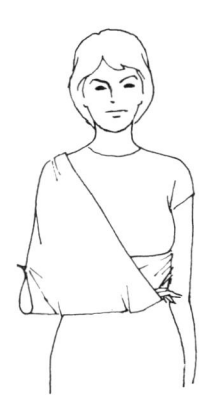

FIGURE 44. SLING. (SEE ALSO FIGURES 25 AND 26, PP. 228–229)

NURSING REFERENCE 19-1
Arm Circumference Measurement

1. Measure circumference:

   - 7 cm above olecranon
   - 11 cm below olecranon

2. Report increases to physician:

   - 0 to 2 cm increase — minimal lymphedema
   - 3 to 6 cm increase — moderate lymphedema
   - 6 cm or greater increase — severe lymphedema

PATIENT EDUCATION SHEET 19-3
Postoperative Exercises

Finger Flexion and Extension

1. Open and close fingers of affected arm.
2. Repeat five times.

Finger Abduction and Adduction

1. Extend fingers of affected arm.
2. Spread them apart as far as possible, and then bring them back together.
3. Repeat five times.

Opposition

1. Extend fingers of affected arm.
2. Touch together thumb and fifth fingers, and then spread them apart.
3. Repeat five times.

Wrist Flexion, Extension, and Rotation

1. Bend wrist forward and backward.
2. Rotate wrist in a circle.
3. Repeat five times.

Supination and Pronation

1. Turn palm down, and then turn palm face up.
2. Repeat five times.

Hand Squeezing

1. Hold a rubber ball or folded washcloth in affected hand.
2. Squeeze the ball tightly, and then release.
3. Repeat five times.

NURSING REFERENCE 19-2
Mastectomy Exercises

1. Patient begins exercise starting at the most comfortable position.
2. Bilateral arm activity is preferred.
3. Fear of pain is lessened by premedication and by having the patient do her own active exercise.
4. Encourage exercises at least four times a day, evenly spaced to prevent exhaustion and pain.
5. Do not expect more shoulder motion than patient was capable of preoperatively.

PATIENT EDUCATION SHEET 19-4
Post-Mastectomy Exercises

Hand Wall Climbing

Position: Standing facing the wall with feet slightly apart and forehead touching the wall (Figure 45)

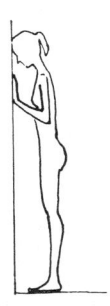

FIGURE 45

1. Place both palms on the wall at shoulder level. Slowly walk your fingers up the wall until incisional pulling or pain occurs. At this point, have someone make a mark indicating your progress (Figure 46).

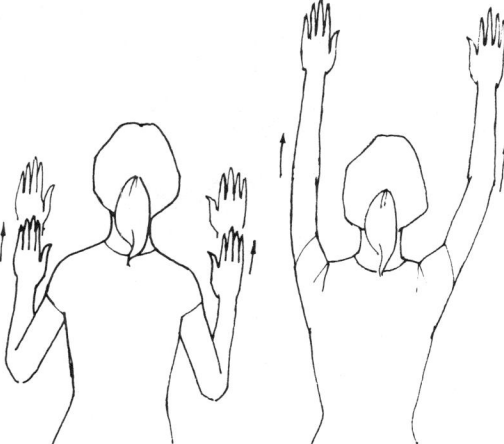

FIGURE 46

286   Site-Specific Protocols

2. Now walk your fingers down the wall to shoulder level. Rest and repeat four more times.

3. You will go higher on succeeding days until both your arms are fully extended.

Clasp, Reach, and Spread

Position: Sitting with hands clasped together

1. Slowly raise your hands in the direction of the top of your head. When you feel your incision begin to pull, *stop* — hold that position and breathe deeply until the pull stops. Continue raising your hands until you reach the top of your head (Figure 47).

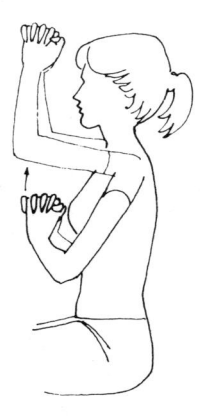

FIGURE 47

Breast Cancer 287

2. Now, slide your hands behind your head to your neck, keeping your head straight (Figures 48 and 49).

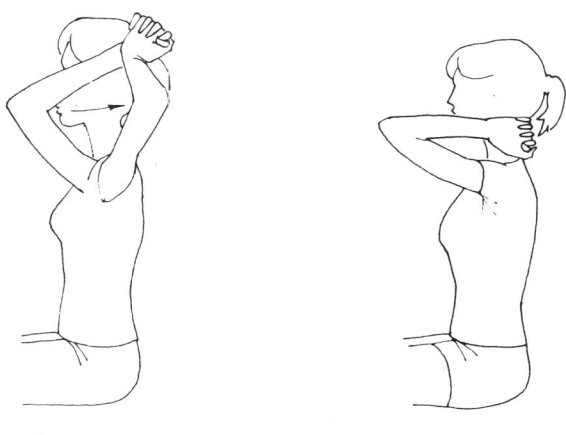

FIGURE 48 **FIGURE 49**

3. Gradually spread your elbows apart. When you feel your incision begin to pull, stop. Hold that position and breathe deeply until the pull stops (Figure 50).

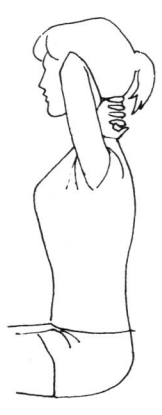

FIGURE 50

4. When your arms are tired, pull your elbows close together and bring your hands back to the top of your head and then down to your lap.

Pulley Exercise

Position: Sitting on the edge of a chair

1. Tie a wooden tongue blade to each end of the rope. Place the rope over a hook above your head.
2. Place one tongue blade in your affected hand. With the uninvolved hand, grasp the other tongue blade and slowly pull your affected arm up (Figure 51).

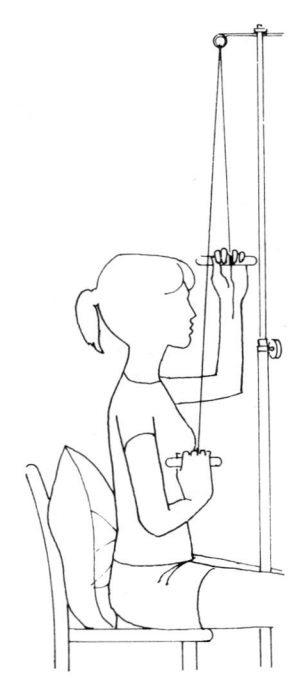

FIGURE 51

Breast Cancer 289

3. When you begin to feel incisional pulling, *stop*. Take deep breaths, and then slowly pull the affected arm up as high as you can (Figure 52). Keep the rope close to your body.
4. Return to the starting position by pulling down with the affected hand until it rests in your lap (Figure 53).

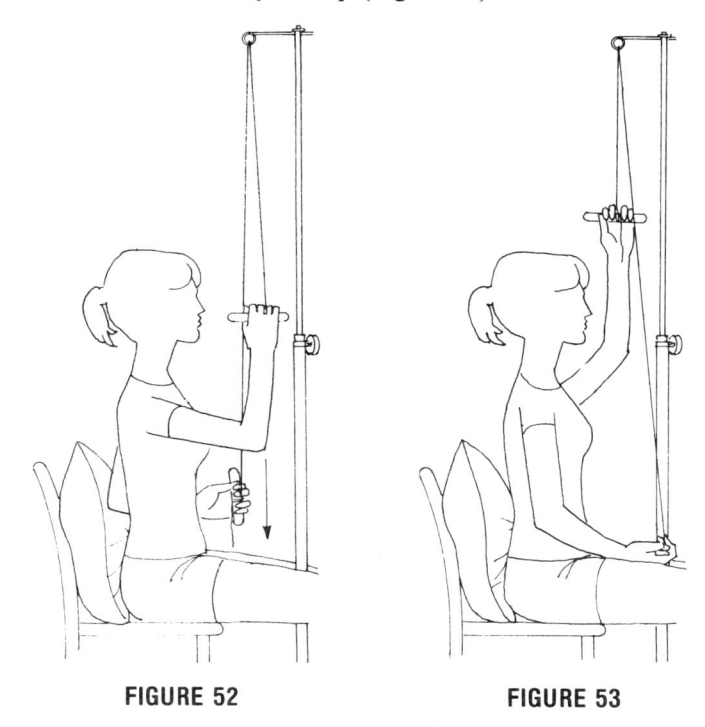

FIGURE 52   **FIGURE 53**

PATIENT EDUCATION SHEET 19-5
Suggestions for Preventing Infection and Swelling of Affected Arm and Hand

Activities at Home*	Suggestions
Sewing	Use thimble; watch out for pinpricks.
Washing dishes	Wear loose-fitting gloves; avoid keeping hand in harsh detergent solution for long periods.
Manicure of hands and cutting of cuticles	Use lanolin-based cream to keep cuticles soft instead of cutting or pricking them.
Gardening	Wear strong work gloves. Let others handle strenuous physical labor.
Baking	Use unaffected arm when reaching into hot oven.
Sunbathing	Use covering across shoulder and arm. Any radiated skin should be protected from sun.
Housework	Let other family members move heavy furniture; avoid activities that require strenuous physical movements; elevate and rest arm if heavy or swollen.
Carrying heavy articles and purse and wearing wrist watch	Use unaffected arm.

*Precaution to be taken in hospital or physician's office: Use unaffected arm for blood pressure readings, injections, intravenous procedures, and blood work.

PATIENT EDUCATION SHEET 19-6
Postural Exercise

1. Stand in front of mirror.
2. Square shoulders by rolling them back, keeping arms at sides.
3. Do this prior to ambulating each time.
4. Do not lean on affected side.

PATIENT EDUCATION SHEET 19-7
Activity Guidelines for Mastectomy Patients

1. Develop good body posture and alignment. Look your best and you will feel your best.//

2. Use both upper extremities when engaging in any tasks. Do not lift, push, or pull more than two pounds the first three weeks. When your incision has healed, do not lift more than one-quarter of your weight. When you do, use good body mechanics so that the stress is distributed over your whole body. Postpone the very stressful activities for approximately three months.

3. Rest between tasks. Your work tolerance and endurance and productivity will be better.

4. Keep up your exercises to maintain full range of motion and muscle tone.

5. Let moderation be the key to your enthusiasm for work and play.

PATIENT EDUCATION SHEET 19-8
Temporary Prosthesis

1. A temporary breast form and bra are sometimes provided by the American Cancer Society's Reach to Recovery volunteer.

2. The fiber-filled prosthesis is lightweight and may be pinned in position directly over the dressing or in the cup of loose bra.

3. For the large-breasted woman, it may be necessary to use a strip of material pinned at the affected cup and panty to prevent the bra from riding up.

PATIENT EDUCATION SHEET 19-9
Permanent Prosthesis Information

Resources for Purchase

1. Reach to Recovery's list of dealers in the area
2. Surgical supply stores
3. Department stores — foundation section
4. Corset shops

Cost

1. Medicare — reimbursable under Part B, with a physician's prescription.
2. Private insurance — usually reimbursable under major medical coverage, with physician's prescription. Check with insurance company for full details.
3. Uncovered cost of prosthesis and special bras are tax deductible. This includes fitting and altering a bra. Obtain a physician's prescription and retain bill.

Shopping Advice

1. Compare styles and prices. Do not automatically assume that a high-priced prosthesis is better than a less expensive model.
2. Try different types of prostheses, comparing comfort, appearance, and fit.
3. Wear a dress that hugs your bustline closely when fitting for a permanent prosthesis. Choose a form that matches your other breast.
4. Bra extenders and shoulder pads may be used to relieve discomfort from the pressure of the bra on the incision.

NURSING REFERENCE 19-3
Self-Help Programs

Reach to Recovery

Description of program

Volunteers from the American Cancer Society's Reach to Recovery Program are former mastectomees who have been trained to do patient visitations. They will visit a patient in the hospital and/or at home.

Procedure for referral

1. Obtain physician consent for Reach to Recovery visit.

2. Contact appropriate local American Cancer Society office with the following information:

   - Patient's name
   - Address
   - Telephone number
   - Age
   - Diagnosis
   - Date and type of surgery
   - Type of medical insurance
   - Patient's bra size

Encore

Description of program

This Young Women's Christian Association program provides postoperative group rehabilitation to help mastectomy patients regain their physical and emotional strength. Program generally consists of floor exercises, pool exercises, and discussion. Instructors are qualified professional women.

Procedure for referral

1. Obtain consent from physician for patient to participate in Encore program.
2. Mastectomy patient can enroll in Encore beginning the third week after surgery.

Chapter 20
COLON CANCER

Preoperative preparation
Alteration in bowel elimination
Potential for injury, perineal wound infection
Potential impairment of skin integrity, related to leakage
Knowledge deficit, odor and gas
Knowledge deficit, colostomy management
Potential impairment of skin integrity, side effects of therapy
Disturbance in self-concept
Sexual dysfunction
Patient Education Sheet 20-1: Pouch Change
Nursing Reference 20-1: Irrigation of Colostomy
Patient Education Sheet 20-2: Appliance for Transverse Colostomy
Patient Education Sheet 20-3: Diet Suggestions for Colostomy Clients
Patient Education Sheet 20-4: Financial Reimbursement for Ostomy Supplies
Patient Education Sheet 20-5: Colostomy Management
Nursing Reference 20-2: Ostomy Club Volunteer Visits

PREOPERATIVE PREPARATION

Evaluation of:

- Best site for stoma placement (enterostomal therapist)
- Activities of daily living ability and limitations

Instruction about:

- Purpose
- How a stoma looks and functions

Introduction to:

- Enterostomal therapist
- Ostomy Club member

NURSING DIAGNOSIS

Alteration in bowel elimination, related to the loss of bowel control secondary to the creation of a colostomy

OUTCOME

Achieves bowel control

INTERVENTIONS

Hospital

1. Immediately after surgery, fit client with appropriate appliance (Patient Education Sheet 20-1).
2. Check appliance seal frequently for signs of leakage.
3. Determine appropriate method (irrigation versus nonirrigation) of attaining bowel control for client based upon:

    - Physical abilities — manual dexterity, mental clarity, loss of a limb, activity tolerance, pre-existing medical conditions
    - Emotional readiness — anxiety level, fears
    - Former bowel pattern
    - Location of ostomy in the colon — clients with transverse/ascending colostomies are not candidates for management by irrigation, as the stools are too liquid and too frequent.

4. Initiate instruction about the appliance that is appropriate for the chosen method of management and the client's manual dexterity.
5. Consult with enterostomal therapist for problems with pouch selection.

Home

1. Evaluate physical and emotional readiness for learning colostomy irrigation. Initiate instruction as appropriate (Nursing Reference 20-1).

2. If nonirrigation method is chosen, assess:

    - Patient's ability to perform pouch changes
    - Suitability of appliance used given the client's life-style

NURSING DIAGNOSIS

Potential for injury, related to perineal wound infection

OUTCOME

Shows no evidence of wound infection

INTERVENTIONS

Hospital

1. Immediately after surgery, inspect perineal wound for bleeding and the presence of drainage catheters.
2. Medicate for pain and evaluate effectiveness.
3. Teach client and family methods of dealing with perineal wound discomfort and its care
   - Sitz baths for cleansing and comfort
   - four-inch-thick foam pad to relieve perineal pressure and discomfort when sitting
   - Positioning
   - Wound irrigation with medicated solutions if wound is open

Home

1. Assess rate of healing; report presence of foul drainage, continued pain, or poor healing to physician.
2. Assess and reinforce client's method of care.
3. Explain that drainage may continue for several weeks.

NURSING DIAGNOSIS

Potential impairment of skin integrity, related to leakage of feces

OUTCOME

Shows no evidence of stoma-related skin problems

INTERVENTIONS

Hospital

1. Use skin barrier under pouch.

2. After removing appliance, examine peristomal skin for signs of irritation:

    - Redness
    - Blistering
    - Excoriation

3. Empty pouch frequently to prevent gas and feces from breaking the appliance seal.

4. Change appliance at the first sign of leakage.

5. Consult with enterostomal therapist for problems with continued leakage.

Home

1. Assess the status of peristomal skin.

2. Determine wear-time of appliance being used. Instruct client to change pouch before pouch begins to leak.

3. Identify factors that may affect wear-time:

   - Activity—type and amount
   - Weight gain or loss
   - Presence of scars or incisions near appliance
   - Climate—temperature and humidity

4. Refer to enterostomal therapist for continued problems with leakage.

NURSING DIAGNOSIS

Knowledge deficit, related to management of odor and gas

OUTCOME

Describes measures to control odor and gas

INTERVENTIONS

Hospital

1. Apply pouch with odor-resistant properties. Check to see that appliance is sealed properly.
2. Refrain from punching holes in pouch to release gas. Use a pouch with a deodorizing charcoal filter if excessive flatulence is a problem.
3. Utilize pouch deodorants and cleansing agents to control odor. Instruct client and family in use.
4. Inform client and family about odor/gas-producing foods to avoid (Patient Education Sheet 20-3).
5. Discuss with physician need for oral medications to reduce flatulence or odor (Mylicon, Derifil, Bismuth subgallate).

Home

1. Assess client's method of applying the pouch and cleaning it, and the pouch's odor-resistant properties.
2. Evaluate dietary habits. Review odor/gas-producing foods.
3. Inform client about availability of external and internal deodorizing agents.

NURSING DIAGNOSIS

Knowledge deficit, related to colostomy management

OUTCOME

Achieves independence in colostomy management

INTERVENTIONS

Hospital

1. Assess client's readiness to learn colostomy care:

    - Physical readiness — manual dexterity, mental clarity, activity tolerance
    - Emotional readiness — anxiety level, acceptance
    - Need for inclusion of family

2. Initiate instruction in colostomy care:

    - Show client stoma, how to cleanse stoma, peristomal skin
    - Teach client how to apply skin barrier and appliance
    - Demonstrate pouch-cleaning technique
    - Review method of obtaining supplies
    - Teach signs of monilial infection; demonstrate use of antimonilial powders under appliance

3. Consult with enterostomal therapist for special problems.

4. Refer to home health agency for reinforcement of instruction.

Home

1. Assess client's management of colostomy:

    - Appliance change technique

- Method of emptying pouch
- Odor/gas control measures

2. Initiate instruction in colostomy irrigation if client is a candidate for this method of management (Nursing Reference 20-1).

3. Review with client instructions for:

    - Bathing (Patient Education Sheet 20-5)
    - Traveling
    - Swimming
    - Handling monilial infections
    - Obtaining supplies (Patient Education Sheet 20-4)

4. Refer to enterostomal therapist for special problems.

NURSING DIAGNOSIS

Potential impairment of skin integrity, related to side effects of chemotherapy and/or radiation therapy

OUTCOMES

Identifies factors that cause skin breakdown
Describes measures to protect skin

INTERVENTIONS

Hospital and Home

1. Review, with client and family, side effects of chemotherapy and/or radiation therapy as they relate to the colostomy:

   - Diarrhea due to radiation or chemotherapy
   - Skin fragility due to radiation

2. Teach client to stop colostomy irrigation until diarrhea ceases and to use skin barrier with an open-end pouch.

3. Obtain order for antidiarrhea medication.

4. Discourage frequent or unnecessary pouch changes.

5. Provide a list of constipating foods (Patient Education Sheet 20-3).

NURSING DIAGNOSIS

Disturbance in self-concept, related to loss of bowel control

OUTCOME

Demonstrates behaviors that indicate reintegration of self-concept

INTERVENTIONS

Hospital

1. Demonstrate competence in colostomy care. Show positive outlook while providing care.
2. Prepare client and family for appearance of stoma.
3. Facilitate verbalization of feelings by sensitivity to verbal and nonverbal cues.
4. Arrange Ostomy Club volunteer visitation.
5. Initiate instruction in self-care.

Home

1. Assess client's ability to manage colostomy care. Continue instruction about daily management (Patient Education Sheet 20-5).
2. Facilitate ventilation of feelings by sensitivity to verbal and nonverbal cues.
3. Counsel client and spouse.
4. Initiate discussion about work. Refer to social worker if job change is needed.

NURSING DIAGNOSIS

Sexual dysfunction, related to change in a body function or impotence

OUTCOME

States sexual relationship is satisfactory

INTERVENTIONS

Hospital

1. Encourage client and spouse/significant other to share feelings about colostomy.
2. Assure client that his/her feelings about fear of rejection, failure, or injury during sexual intimacy are normal.
3. Teach the client ways to increase sexual attractiveness:

   - Use pouch cover
   - Empty pouch or dressing if needed

4. For males, reinforce physician's explanations about impotence and the availability of penile prostheses.

Home

1. Initiate discussion about sexuality with client and spouse/significant other.
2. Review ways to increase sexual attractiveness.
3. Initiate referrals to facilitate acceptance:

   - Ostomy Club
   - Sexual therapist

4. Encourage male clients to discuss penile prosthesis with physician.

PATIENT EDUCATION SHEET 20-1
Pouch Change

Supplies Needed

- Open-end pouch
- Skin barrier
- External deodorant

Technique

1. Remove old pouch (Figure 54).

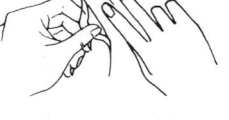

FIGURE 54

2. Examine skin for signs of irritation. Check stoma for color, size, and shape.
3. Cut or enlarge opening in skin barrier to fit around stoma snugly. Cut opening in pouch slightly larger than opening in skin barrier (Figure 55).

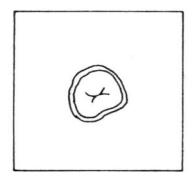

FIGURE 55

4. Cleanse stoma and skin with antiseptic solution or soap and water. Dry well.
5. Saturate a small piece of tissue with deodorant. Insert in pouch.
6. Apply skin barrier and then apply pouch.

NURSING REFERENCE 20-1
Irrigation of Colostomy

Care

1. Provide patient with pamphlet on colostomy management and review pamphlet prior to instruction on irrigation.

2. Evaluate readiness for learning:

   - Physical readiness
   - Ability to sit for 30 minutes with minimal discomfort
   - Absence of physical disabilities
   - Emotional readiness

3. Allow patient to assume as much of his or her own care as possible:

   - Day 1 — instruct with patient assisting.
   - Day 2 — patient does procedure with assistance.
   - Day 3 — patient does procedure with prompting only as needed.
   - Day 4 — Patient does procedure independently.
   - (Modify plan as necessary.)

Supplies Needed

   Colostomy irrigation set containing:

- Cone tip or *soft* flexible catheter with shield
- Calibrated water container
- One-handed regulating clamp
- Plastic irrigating sleeve
- Adjustable belt
- Clips
- Water-soluble lubricant
- Pouch and skin barrier

Technique

1. Fill water container with 1½ quarts lukewarm water.
2. Remove pouch from stoma. Observe stoma and examine skin for irritation.
3. Position irrigating sleeve and fasten snugly with belt.
4. Lubricate catheter or cone tip. With water running slowly, insert catheter or tip into stoma, using a rotating in-and-out motion.
5. Instill one-half to one quart of fluid over a three- to five-minute period.
6. If cramping occurs:

    - Shut off water.
    - Instruct patient to take deep breaths.
    - Check amount of fluid instilled.
    - Instill water more slowly when cramps subside.

7. Remove catheter or cone tip. Clip top of sleeve closed.
8. Allow 30 to 45 minutes for colostomy to empty completely. When drainage has stopped, remove sleeve.

PATIENT EDUCATION SHEET 20-2
Appliance for Transverse Colostomy

Supplies

- Open-end pouch with odor-ban properties
- Skin barrier
- External deodorant
- Paper tape
- Clamp

Technique

1. Remove old pouch (Figure 56). Wipe stoma clean of stool with toilet tissue. Examine skin for signs of irritation.

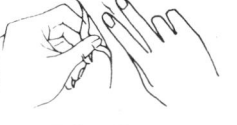

FIGURE 56

2. Cut or enlarge opening in skin barrier so that it is exactly the size of the stoma. Cut an opening in the pouch that is larger than the stoma (Figure 57).

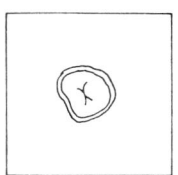

FIGURE 57

3. Cleanse stoma and skin with mild soap and water or antiseptic solution. (Showering is possible when incisions have healed.)
4. Apply skin barrier and then pouch.
5. Saturate a small piece of tissue with deodorant and place in pouch.
6. Reinforce adhesive edges of pouch with strips of paper tape in a picture-frame fashion (Figure 58).

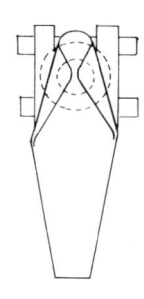

FIGURE 58

Care

1. Provide patient with booklet on colostomy management and review it with patient.
2. Change appliance twice weekly.
3. Empty pouch when half-full to prevent weight from pulling it off.
4. Rinse pouch out with cold water at least once daily (Figure 59). Insert a fresh piece of deodorant-saturated tissue at that time.

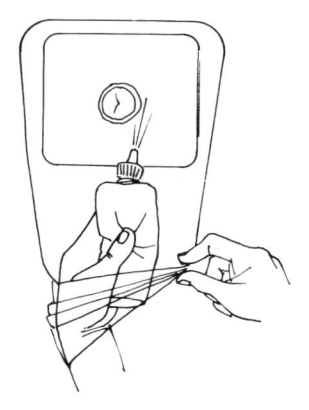

FIGURE 59

5. Irrigations are not recommended since spillage of stool continues in spite of irrigation.
6. Showering is possible.

PATIENT EDUCATION SHEET 20-3
Diet Suggestions for Colostomy Clients

Purpose

The diet for persons with a colostomy is designed to prevent problems with colostomy management. The diet should be well balanced, with new foods introduced one at a time. Foods that previously caused problems for the client will most likely continue to be troublesome.

Odor-Causing Foods

- Beans
- Highly spiced foods
- Onions
- Legumes
- Cabbage
- Eggs
- Certain cheeses
- Asparagus

Constipating foods

- Apple juice
- Bananas

Gas-Producing Foods

- Cauliflower
- Beans
- Broccoli
- Cabbage
- Onions
- Legumes
- Highly spiced foods
- Carbonated drinks
- Beer (has been known to cause diarrhea and gas)

PATIENT EDUCATION SHEET 20-4
Financial Reimbursement for Ostomy Supplies

Medicare

Eighty percent of the cost of ostomy equipment and supplies is reimbursable after payment of the usual yearly deductible.

1. Obtain physician prescription for equipment and supplies.
2. Obtain appropriate form from the Social Security office and submit bills.

Public Welfare Office

One hundred percent of the cost of ostomy equipment and supplies is reimbursable.

1. Obtain physician prescription for equipment and supplies.
2. Contact social worker if dealer does not have a reimbursement agreement with the welfare office.

Private Insurance Companies

Eighty percent of the cost of ostomy equipment and supplies is usually reimbursable under major medical benefits.

1. Obtain physician prescription for equipment and supplies.
2. Contact insurance company for appropriate forms.

Taxable Deductions

Uncovered costs are deductible at income tax time.

1. Obtain physician prescription for equipment and supplies.
2. Retain bills for documentation of payment.

PATIENT EDUCATION SHEET 20-5
Colostomy Management

Bathing

1. Tub baths or showers are possible when the abdominal incision has healed.
2. Bathing may be done with or without a pouch covering the stoma.
3. Soap and water cleansing of the stoma and surrounding skin is essential for odor control.
4. Any type of bath soap is satisfactory; special soaps are not necessary

Travel

1. Irrigation equipment should be checked. Replace all worn parts.
2. A supply of disposable security pouches and a skin barrier sufficient for use during the trip should be ordered.
3. Spillage may occur even with a well-regulated colostomy because of rapid time changes.
4. It is safe to irrigate in any country with water that is safe to *drink*.
5. Diarrhea may result from a change in diet or even from bacteria. Request an effective antidiarrheal medication from the doctor.
6. It is a good idea to hand carry supplies so that stray luggage does not create problems.
7. Keep a disposable security pouch in a handbag or in a pocket for use in emergencies.

Clothing

1. Clothing worn before surgery is still suitable.
2. The stoma is not visible through clothing.

3. Tight girdles or those with rigid boning may irritate the stoma and cause bleeding.

Sports

1. Swimming is possible.

   - Choose bathing dress that is comfortable.
   - Cover the stoma with gauze and paper tape; alternatively, a pouch may be worn.

2. Physical contact sports should be avoided until the doctor permits this type of activity.

NURSING REFERENCE 20-2
Ostomy Club Volunteer Visits

Description of Program

Volunteers from the local ostomy association are available for preoperative and postoperative visitations to the ostomy patient. Volunteers are ostomates who have been trained to make these visits. Age and sex-matching of volunteer and patient are attempted.

Procedure for Referral

1. Obtain physician approval for ostomy volunteer visit.
2. Call the local American Cancer Society office for the nearest ostomy club in the area. Provide information regarding the patient's name, address, age, and surgical procedure, for use by the visitation chairman.

Chapter 21
BLADDER CANCER

Alteration in pattern of urinary elimination
Knowledge deficit, ileal conduit care
Potential impairment of skin integrity
Knowledge deficit, odor
Disturbance in self-concept
Sexual dysfunction
Patient Education Sheet 21-1: Ileal Conduit—Temporary Pouch Change
Patient Education Sheet 21-2: Application of a Permanent Urinary Appliance
Patient Education Sheet 21-3: Ileal Conduit Management

NURSING DIAGNOSIS

Alteration is pattern of urinary elimination, related to loss of urinary control secondary to creation of a urinary diversion

OUTCOME

Achieves urinary continence

INTERVENTIONS

Hospital

1. Immediately after surgery:

   - Fit with disposable pouch, using a skin barrier
   - Observe stoma appearance—color, size, bleeding

2. Check appliance seal frequently for signs of leakage.

3. Discuss with client the choice between a permanent reusable or a disposable appliance based upon:

   - Manual dexterity
   - Cost versus time saved
   - Type of stoma—protruding versus flush or retracted

4. Involve enterostomal therapist if stoma problems are apparent:

   - Flush, retracted stoma
   - Poor placement—near incision, bony prominences, or body skin folds

5. Initiate instruction about appropriate appliance.

Home

1. Assess client's ability to change appliance.
2. Refer to enterostomal therapist for fitting of a permanent reusable appliance if client chooses to use this type of appliance.
3. Assess appliance length-of-wear time. If less than 2–3 days with a satisfactory stoma, re-evaluate client's method of appliance application and pouch-emptying practices.

NURSING DIAGNOSIS

Knowledge deficit, related to ileal conduit care

OUTCOME

Achieves independence in care of ileal conduit

INTERVENTIONS

Hospital

1. Assess client's readiness to learn ileal conduit care:

    - Physical readiness — manual dexterity, mental clarity, activity tolerance
    - Emotional readiness — anxiety level, acceptance
    - Need for inclusion of family

2. Initiate instruction in ileal conduit care:

    - Show client stoma, how to cleanse stoma and peristomal skin
    - Teach client how to apply skin barrier and appliance (Patient Education Sheet 21-1)
    - Demonstrate method of emptying pouch
    - Review method of obtaining supplies
    - Teach signs of monilial infection

3. Consult with enterostomal therapist for special problems.

4. Refer to home health agency for reinforcement of instruction.

Home

1. Assess client's management of ileal conduit:

- Appliance change technique
- Method of emptying pouch
- Odor control measures

2. Initiate instruction on use of permanent reusable appliance if client chooses this method (Patient Education Sheet 21-2).

3. Review with client, instructions for:

    - Dealing with monilial infection
    - Obtaining supplies (Patient Education Sheet 20-4)
    - Bathing (Patient Education Sheet 21-3)
    - Traveling
    - Swimming

4. Refer to enterostomal therapist for special problems.

NURSING DIAGNOSIS

Potential impairment of skin integrity, related to leakage of urine and/or skin irritants

OUTCOMES

Identifies factors that lead to skin breakdown
Describes measures to prevent and manage peristomal skin problems

INTERVENTIONS

Hospital

1. Observe peristomal skin for signs of breakdown at times of pouch change:

    - Redness
    - Blistering
    - Excoriation

2. Protect peristomal skin by:

    - Using a skin barrier under the appliance
    - Cutting an appropriate-sized opening in the skin barrier and appliance (leave no more than one-eighth inch of peristomal skin exposed)

3. Teach client and family common causes of peristomal skin irritation:

    - Ill-fitting appliance
    - Sensitivity to materials in appliance pouch, skin barrier, tapes
    - Warmth and humidity
    - Chemical irritants — soaps, solvents

- Mechanical irritants — pressure from belts, friction
- Monilial infection

4. Teach client and family ways to deal with causes of irritation:

    - Use of a properly fitted appliance with skin barrier
    - Correct method of cleansing peristomal skin
    - Patch testing of skin barriers and adhesives if skin is especially sensitive
    - Use of antimonilial powders or creams

5. Involve enterostomal therapist for problems with skin sensitivity or persistent skin irritation.

Home

1. Assess fit of appliance. Refer to enterostomal therapist for re-fitting of permanent appliance faceplate if more than one-eighth inch of peristomal skin is exposed.
2. Re-instruct regarding skin care.
3. If a permanent, reusable appliance is used, instruct regarding long-term problems related to improper appliance care.

    - Hyperplasia — overgrowth of skin related to a too-large faceplate opening
    - Alkaline encrustations — white crystalline deposits on peristomal skin due to alkaline urine and a too-large faceplate opening
    - Stomal irritation related to build-up of salts around faceplate opening with poor cleaning techniques

4. Encourage visit to enterostomal therapist at least once yearly.

NURSING DIAGNOSIS

Knowledge deficit, related to odor

OUTCOME

Describes measures to control odor

INTERVENTIONS

Hospital

1. Explain that infection is common cause of odor. Teach measures to prevent urinary tract infection:

   - Liberal fluid intake
   - Acidification of urine by use of vitamin C tablets (approximately 1 gm/day).

2. Teach client and family appropriate appliance care techniques.

Home

1. Review appliance care and cleansing instructions.
2. Assess client's fluid intake and acidity of urine using Nitrazene paper.
3. Check permanent appliance parts for signs of over-use or improper cleaning. Consider switch to disposable appliance if a permanent reusable appliance is cause of odor.

NURSING DIAGNOSIS

Disturbance in self-concept, related to loss of urinary control

OUTCOME

Demonstrates behaviors which indicate reintegration of self-concept

INTERVENTIONS

Hospital

1. Demonstrate competence in ostomy care. Show positive outlook while providing care.
2. Ensure continence through use of a postoperative appliance (Patient Education Sheet 21-1).
3. Prepare client and spouse for appearance of stoma.
4. Facilitate verbalization of feelings by sensitivity to verbal and nonverbal cues.
5. Arrange Ostomy Club volunteer visitation.
6. Initiate teaching about self-care.

Home

1. Reinforce patient's ability to perform self-care.
2. Initiate and continue discussion about management of ileal conduit in daily living (Patient Education Sheet 21-3).
3. Arrange ostomy volunteer visit if not already done (Nursing Reference 20-2).
4. Initiate discussion about work. Refer to social worker if job change is needed.

NURSING DIAGNOSIS

Sexual dysfunction, related to change in body function or impotence

OUTCOME

States sexual relationship is satisfactory

INTERVENTIONS

Hospital

1. Encourage client and spouse/significant other to share feelings about the urinary diversion.
2. Assure client that his/her feelings about fear of rejection, failure, or injury during sexual intimacy are normal.
3. Teach the client ways to increase sexual attractiveness:

    - Use pouch cover
    - Empty pouch prior to sexual activity
    - Change pouch if needed

4. For males, reinforce physician's explanations about impotence and the availability of penile prostheses.

Home

1. Initiate discussion about sexuality with spouse/significant other.
2. Review ways to increase sexual attractiveness.
3. Initiate referrals to facilitate acceptance:

    - Ostomy Club
    - Sexual therapist

4. Encourage male clients to discuss penile prosthesis with physician.

PATIENT EDUCATION SHEET 21-1
Ileal Conduit—Temporary Pouch Change

Supplies Needed

- Urinary postoperative pouch with drain tip
- Skin barrier (optional—spray, gel, or methyl cellulose wafer preferred)

Technique

1. Remove old pouch. Examine skin and stoma for signs for irritation.
2. Cut opening in the pouch that is one-eighth inch larger than the stoma all around. An exact size opening will cut and irritate the stoma.
3. Cleanse skin with mild soap and water or antiseptic solution.
4. Apply skin barrier if desired, covering stoma with gauze or rolled-up tissue wick.
5. Apply pouch.
6. Reinforce pouch edges with paper tape in picture-frame fashion.

Care

1. Change pouch every two to three days.
2. Empty pouch when half-full to prevent weight from pulling it off.

PATIENT EDUCATION SHEET 21-2
Application of a Permanent Urinary Appliance

Supplies

- One pouch
- One faceplate
- One locking ring or elastic band
- One double-faced adhesive
- One stoma guide strip
- Scissors
- Soap
- Washcloths
- Adhesive remover
- Skin barrier (gel, spray, or methyl cellulose wafer preferred)

Technique

1. Assemble permanent appliance. Remove paper backing from one side of double-faced adhesive and apply to faceplate. Remove second paper backing. Insert a stoma guide strip.

2. If using a doubled-faced adhesive and gel or spray skin barrier:

    - Take off pouch using adhesive remover.
    - Examine skin for any redness or irritation.
    - Rinse off soap completely.
    - Dry skin thoroughly.
    - Apply light coat of skin barrier. Allow to dry completely.
    - Apply appliance.
    - Reinforce adhesive edges with a paper tape in a picture-frame fashion.

3. If using methyl cellulose wafer:

   - Gently peel off pouch.
   - Examine skin for any redness or irritation.
   - Cut a hole in the wafer to fit stoma exactly.
   - Wash skin and stoma with soap.
   - Rinse off soap completely.
   - Dry skin thoroughly.
   - Apply wafer.
   - Apply the pouch.
   - Reinforce adhesive edges of pouch with paper tape in a picture-frame fashion.

4. Make a solution of appliance-cleaning agent and water. Empty used pouch and rinse with water and then soak in solution. Check for sandy build-up in opening of faceplate. If this is present, wash opening with a brush. Rinse out pouch and allow to dry on hanger.

Care

1. Change appliance at least once weekly.
2. Empty pouch when half-full.

PATIENT EDUCATION SHEET 21-3
Ileal Conduit Management

Bathing

1. Tub baths or showers are possible when the abdominal incision has healed.
2. Bathing is done with the pouch on, except for those times when bathing and pouch changing coincide. At those times, it is possible to bathe without a pouch on.
3. Soap and water cleansing of the stoma and surrounding skin during a pouch change is essential for odor control.
4. Any type of bath soap is satisfactory—special soaps are not necessary.

Travel

1. Check appliance parts, replace all worn parts. It is often very difficult to find replacements one is familiar with in a strange city.
2. Take along a spare appliance and enough double-faced adhesive tape discs for the duration of the trip.
3. Keep one or two adhesive tape discs in a handbag or pocket for use during emergencies.
4. *Plan* when pouch changes should be made. Do not postpone a pouch change or an embarrassing leak may occur.

Clothing

1. The appliance should *not* be visible under the usual clothing. If it is, the enterostomal therapist should be consulted for an appliance that is less visible.
2. Tight girdles or those with rigid boning may irritate the stoma and cause bleeding.

Bladder Cancer

Sports

1. Swimming is possible.

    - Choose bathing dress that is comfortable.
    - Reinforce adhesive edges of pouch with paper tape to make it waterproof.

2. Physical contact sports should be avoided until the doctor permits this type of activity.

    - Empty pouch before engaging in activity.
    - Reinforce adhesive edges pouch with *new* pieces of paper tape.
    - After the activity, check the position of the appliance over the stoma. Change the appliance if it is not centered directly over the stoma.

Chapter 22
PROSTATE CANCER

Preoperative preparation
Fluid volume deficit, bleeding
Alteration in pattern of urinary elimination
Sexual dysfunction related to impotence
Patient Education Sheet 22-1: Perineal Exercises

PREOPERATIVE PREPARATION

Discussion with patient and spouse about:

- Possibility of incontinence

Instruct in:

- Perineal exercises

NURSING DIAGNOSIS

Fluid volume deficit, related to hemorrhage from the prostatic fossa

OUTCOME

Shows evidence of minimal bleeding

INTERVENTIONS

Hospital

1. Observe for:

   - Bleeding, blood clots from foley catheter — note color of drainage, viscosity
   - Reports of needing to void, bladder spasms

2. Follow physician's orders for foley traction, continuous bladder irrigation.

3. Instruct client to:

   - Avoid straining during defecation
   - Include natural laxative foods in diet
   - Use stool softners as prescribed

Home

1. Instruct client to report changes in urine color, character.
2. Teach client to curtail strenuous activities, lifting.

NURSING DIAGNOSIS

Alteration in pattern of urinary elimination: incontinence, related to inability to control micturation

OUTCOMES

Achieves urinary control
Identifies ways to manage incontinence

INTERVENTIONS

Hospital

1. Explain reason for incontinence—removal of internal sphincter.
2. Teach client perineal exercises (Patient Education Sheet 22-1).
3. Apply and teach about the use of incontinence appliances.

Home

1. Assess extent of urinary control achieved by perineal exercises (Patient Education Sheet 22-1).
2. Determine efficiency of incontinence appliance.
3. Help client deal with frustration if incontinence becomes permanent.

NURSING DIAGNOSIS

Sexual dysfunction related to impotence

OUTCOME

Describes alternative ways to achieve satisfactory sexual relationship

INTERVENTIONS

Hospital

1. Assess readiness of client to discuss concerns regarding sexuality.
2. Encourage interaction between client and spouse about sexuality.
3. Explain about the availability of several penile prostheses.
4. Refer to Self-Concept and Sexuality Protocols (Chapters 10 and 11).

Home

1. Provide opportunity for client to discuss feelings about his sexuality.
2. Refer to sexual therapist as needed.
3. Encourage client to discuss penile prosthesis surgery with the physician.

PATIENT EDUCATION SHEET 22-1
Perineal Exercise

Purpose

To strengthen the urethral sphincter mechanism and to increase tone of perineal muscle

Exercise

1. Relax body. Tighten or squeeze anus as if to prevent defecation, and then tighten perineal muscles as if to prevent urination.
2. Keep hands on abdomen to ensure that abdominal muscles are not contracted.
3. Repeat 20 times every hour while awake. If done correctly, the penis will react with each squeeze.

Chapter 23
STOMACH CANCER

Alteration in nutrition, less than body requirements
Knowledge deficit
Alteration in bowel elimination

NURSING DIAGNOSIS

Alteration in nutrition, to less than body requirements, related to discomfort from gastric atony or dumping syndrome

OUTCOME

Identifies measures to optimize food intake

INTERVENTIONS

1. Explain reasons for:

   - Dumping syndrome
   - Gastric atony

2. Discuss signs and symptoms of dumping syndrome

   - Profuse perspiration
   - Weakness, faintness
   - Nausea and vomiting
   - Palpitations
   - Epigastric fullness

3. Teach patient to:

   - Eat small, frequent meals
   - Restrict concentrated carbohydrates
   - Incorporate increased amounts of protein as tolerated
   - Add fat only as tolerated
   - Separate solids from liquids

4. Consult with dietitian regarding progression and modification of diet.
5. Monitor weight closely.
6. Stress importance of continuing vitamins and iron supplementation.

NURSING DIAGNOSIS

Knowledge deficit, related to jejunostomy management

OUTCOME

Demonstrates ability to manage jejunostomy care

INTERVENTIONS

1. Reinforce explanation about jejunostomy being a temporary adjunct to gastrectomy.
2. Teach client/family about jejunostomy feedings:

   - Use of enteral pump to infuse feeding at a constant rate
   - Gradually increasing strength (concentration) of feeding
   - Changing from constant to intermittent feedings when client can tolerate greater volumes

3. Review with client and family jejunostomy tube care

   - Care of skin around catheter
   - Infection at catheter site
   - Handling of catheter occlusion

4. Consult with dietitian for problems related to formula intolerance.

NURSING DIAGNOSIS

Alteration in bowel elimination: constipation, related to low residue diet or enteral feedings

OUTCOME

Verbalizes understanding of reason for decreased frequency of stools

INTERVENTIONS

1. Assess for hardening of stools and decrease in the usual patterns of bowel elimination.
2. Re-evaluate client's understanding of low residue formula and its potential for decreasing bowel movements.
3. Encourage increasing amount of water and fluids via jejunostomy catheter.
4. Consult with physician regarding medications that contribute to constipation.
5. Confer with dietitian to determine need for change in formula for feedings.